Aromatherapy Solutions

essential 3

100% Pure Therapeutic-Quality
Essential Oils

THIRD EDITION

A special thanks to Lakita, Joni, and Chris.

For information about Essential 3 products and their use, please contact:

ESSENTIAL 3
541-858-3313
aroma@essentialthree.com
www.essentialthree.com

Book and cover design by
Chris Molé Design

PRINTED IN THE USA

TABLE OF CONTENTS

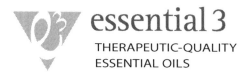

essential 3
THERAPEUTIC-QUALITY
ESSENTIAL OILS

ESSENTIAL 3 provides therapeutic-quality essential oils at affordable prices. We define therapeutic-quality as being free of pesticides, synthetics, stretching, and any adulteration. In addition, the chemical constituents are in the required percentile range necessary for the essential oil to be considered therapeutic.

Our essential oils are 100% pure and authentic. An independent lab tests all of our oils. A Ph.D. chemist compiles the test results and provides *Certificate of Analysis* evaluation and documentation. These reports are available to our customers.

We purchase in large quantities and bottle and label ourselves. This helps us keep the essential oils we offer affordable and of consistent quality.

If you have any questions about ℮³ essential oils or how to use them, please contact us. We have clinical aromatherapists on staff to help you. If you are looking for an essential oil that is not listed, please inquire as we stock a variety of unique essential oils to meet the needs of blenders, perfumers, and aromatherapists.

*Warm regards from all of us at **Essential 3***

REACH US AT:
Customer Service / Order: 541-858-3313
Email: aroma@essentialthree.com
Fax: 866-279-1989
Website: www.essentialthree.com

This material is not intended as a substitute for consulting with your physician or other health care provider. Any attempt to diagnose or treat an illness should be done under the direction of a health-care professional.

Aromatherapy: The use of natural, aromatic substances, known as essential oils, to enhance the well-being of body, mind, and spirit.

(This statement has not been evaluated by the FDA. No information provided is intended to diagnose, treat, cure or prevent any disease.)

General Essential Oil Information

Why Essential Oils are Beneficial?

Essential oils offer an effective holistic approach to support health and well-being for our body, mind and spirit. Each essential oil has a unique pharmacological effect, such as antibacterial, antiviral, rejuvenating, calming, anti-inflammatory, diuretic, vasodilator, sedative, adrenal stimulating, to name a few.

What is an Essential Oil?

Essential oils are concentrated, hydrophobic liquids, containing volatile aroma compounds, extracted from plants (seeds, resin, blossoms, fruits, berries, bark, leaves, roots, peel, flowers, or the entire plant). "Essential oils may contain hundreds of chemical constituents that are responsible for cellular energy production, growth, attraction of pollinating insects, cell repair and defense against viruses, bacteria, fungi, and predatory insects" * The oils are produced in special plant cells, from the sun, the air, soil, and water.

How do we get Essential Oils?

Essential oils are procured from the plant by various methods of extraction; which include, Water or Steam Distillation, (the most common form), Hydro Diffusion, Solvent extractions, CO_2 (Carbon Dioxide), Cold Expression, Enfleurage, and Maceration. Hydrosols are the by-product of the distillation process.

What is Aromatherapy?

It is the controlled use of essential oils to maintain and promote physical, psychological, and emotional balance.

What is Clinical Aromatherapy?

Clinical Aromatherapy is the therapeutic use and application of genuine and authentic plant derived essential oils for the support of patients (clients) health and well-being.

Aromatherapy combines well with many complementary modalities: massage therapy, energy work, Reiki, Healing Touch, acupuncture, acupressure, chiropractic, cranial sacral, reflexology, gemstone therapy, breath work, yoga, guided visual imagery, clinical hypnotherapy, and hydrotherapy.

What Aromatherapy is not...

The term Aromatherapy is trendy and fashionable and it is important to realize that it is NOT just smelly stuff! It is not candles, dish soap, air freshener or garbage bags scented with synthetic fragrance. Do not be misled.

Chemistry of essential oils:

Essential oils are mixtures of aromatic molecules built from three basic elements: carbon, hydrogen and oxygen. A few may also contain sulfur and nitrogen.

* Raphael J. d'Angelo M.D. – Fundamentals of Aromatic Medicine p.1

How Essential Oils Affect a Person via Inhalation and Skin Absorption

Inhalation:

Olfactory absorption: Olfaction is the sense of smell. Smell is the least understood of all our senses, but it is known that it is 10,000 times more sensitive than taste. Scent is the key that opens up the mind to the memory. Aromas enter via the nasal cavity and are received by thousands of olfactory nerves and the tiny essential oil molecules react with the specific nerve receptors and are sent directly to the limbic system.

The Limbic System: The limbic system includes the hippocampus, amygdala, anterior thalamic nuclei, septum, habenula, limbic cortex and fornix. It supports a variety of functions, including emotion, behavior, motivation, long-term memory, and olfaction. When we first smell an aroma, neural signals go to the amygdala which interprets the emotional significance the aroma. In other words, an aroma can trigger emotions which then results in a behavior appropriate to the external circumstances; i.e. aromas can help to stimulate the "fight or flight" survival response or help to facilitate calm, supporting the maintenance of homeostasis in our body systems.

Sinus and Lung Absorption: The respiratory system consists of the nasal passages, larynx, pharynx, trachea and lungs, which in turn consist of the bronchial tubes, the bronchioles and the alveoli sacs. It is here, in the sacs and via the nasal mucosa that the essential oil constituents pass into the bloodstream and through the blood brain barrier, entering the central nervous system. Essential oil molecules behave like pharmaceuticals in terms of their distribution, metabolism and elimination via the liver, kidneys, integumentary and the respiratory system.

Skin absorption:

Skin, the largest organ of the body, is composed of three parts; the epidermis, the dermis, and the hypodermis. It is responsible for excretion, respiration and protection of underlying tissues. The skin also supports a network of nerve endings whose function is to relay sensations to the brain, such as cold, heat and pain.

The small molecular structure of essential oils and their affinity to the skins oil (sebum) allow certain constituents to penetrate into the layers of epidermis. Once the essential oil constituents have passed the epidermis they enter the dermis (capillaries, lymph vessels, nerves, sweat and oil glands, collagen and follicles). The molecules are then carried from the capillaries into the blood stream where they are circulated throughout the body; elimination occurs via sweat glands and normal body functions.

Essential Oil Safety Guidelines

Essential oils are concentrated, active, plant extracts; thus care and responsibility must be taken with their use. The following are standard, recommended safety guidelines for using essential oils.

1. Keep essential oils out of reach of children.

2. Essential oils are intended for external use. (Do not take essential oils internally unless under the direction of a qualified health professional.)

3. Dilute essential oils in a carrier before they are applied to the skin.

4. Test for sensitivities. Wash and dry an area on the inside of elbow. Apply the diluted oil, preferably cover and leave for 24 hours. If redness or irritation occurs apply a vegetable oil, then wash with soap and water.

5. Avoid essential oil contact with eyes, mucous membranes, and other sensitive areas.

6. Keep essential oils away from open flames.

7. Dilute essential oils in a carrier before adding them to your bath. (Essential oils do not dilute in water due to their hydrophobic nature.) See Methods of Using Essential Oils, page xi.

8. Certain essential oils, especially those from the citrus family, can cause photosensitivity—discoloration and/or irritation of the skin when exposed to ultraviolet light. These essential oils should not be used in products that remain on the skin (such as in a lotion or perfume) at least 12 hours before being in direct sunlight, using sunlamps or tanning beds.

9. Certain essential oils have very strong characteristics, such as Cinnamon, Oregano, Thyme ct. thymol, Wintergreen, and Clove. Use in a 1-3% dilution and for short periods of time.

10. Keep a carrier oil readily available when using essential oils. In case of skin irritation, apply the carrier directly to the affected area. If no carrier is available, flush area with water for 15 minutes.

11. Do not use essential oils rich in menthol, such as peppermint with children under 3 years of age.

12. Overexposure or sensitivity to an essential oil through inhalation may result in nausea, headache, emotional unease or a "spacey" feeling. Getting some fresh air and drinking water will help to ease these symptoms.

13. Store essential oils tightly closed in dark, glass bottles, away from heat and light.

14. Use only pure essential oils from plants; GC, MS, FID tested to insure quality.

This material is not intended as a substitute for consulting with your physician or other health care provider. Any attempt to diagnose or treat an illness should be done under the direction of a health-care professional.

Aromatherapy: The use of natural, aromatic substances, known as essential oils, to enhance the well-being of body, mind, and spirit.

(This statement has not been evaluated by the FDA. No information provided is intended to diagnose, treat, cure or prevent any disease.)

Precautions and Contraindications

Pregnancy and Lactation
Consult your health care professional before using essential oils during pregnancy, labor, and lactation.

The use of essential oils during pregnancy and lactation is a controversial issue in the aromatherapy field. According to most aromatherapy references, there are essential oils to be avoided. It is recommended that anyone who is pregnant or lactating and intends to use essential oils, consult with their physician and conduct their own research, using a variety of sources, to determine personal guidelines for use.

Babies and Children
Consult your health care professional before using essential oils with babies and children. It is important to ensure proper essential oil selection, dilution, and method, specific to your child.

"A baby's liver and kidneys are not fully functioning until after two years of age and are still developing up to the age of seven, making their ability to process and remove essential oils from the body inhibited." *Fiona Cuthbert O'Meara, RN, Aromatherapist*

Elderly or Frail
When using essential oils with the elderly or frail, it is important to use in a 1-5% dilution.

Medical Conditions
If you have serious health issues consult with your health care professional before using essential oils. If you have or have had estrogen-dependent tumors, it is recommended that you avoid phytoestrogenic essential oils such as Anise, Clary Sage, Fennel, Angelica, and Tarragon. For more information refer to *Clinical Aromatherapy* by Jane Buckle.

Allergy Prone / Sensitive Skin
If you are allergy prone or have sensitive skin, it is recommended that you test an essential oil before using it.

Wash and dry an area on the inside of your elbow. Apply a drop of the essential oil and cover it with a strip bandage. Leave in place for twenty-four hours. Take the bandage off and assess your skin. If there is no reaction, there should not be an allergy or sensitivity to the essential oil. If there is swelling or irritation do not use the essential oil, and clean the area by applying a carrier oil and then washing with soap and water. Rinse well and pat dry.

Homeopathic Remedies
If you are taking a homeopathic remedy, essential oils may negate its effect. Those especially indicated are Eucalyptus, Peppermint, and Rosemary.

"What interests me as a neuropsychopharmacologist is the way essential oils pass easily through the skin and travel efficiently thought the body in a similar fashion to hormones and neuropeptides. The oils find receptor sites on cells to act as catalysts for change within the cell metabolism. The oils are an outside influence on the vital communication network taking place between the nervous, endocrine, and immune systems in the mind-body, what I've called the bodymind. The ability of essential oils to harmonize emotion, raise out spirits and eliminate microbial infections has made them extremely precious and highly sought after throughout our human history. Only recently have the molecular cellular mechanisms of these powerful herbal preparations been studied by scientists.

Integrative medicine holds the great promise of helping us to understand the unity of the mind and body in order to achieve the greatest state of health possible."

Candace B. Pert, PhD
July 17, 2009
Potomac, Maryland
Taken from her introduction to
Awaken to Healing Fragrance
author Elizabeth Anne Jones

Methods of Using Essential Oils

The methods and number of drops described below are general guidelines for healthy adult use. Individual sensitivities, the desired results, and the characteristics of the essential oil(s) used must all be considered. Adjust methods and proportions accordingly.

Add to Products: Essential oils can be added to pre-made, fragrance-free products to enhance their performance. Add 4-8 drops to 2 ounces of facial moisturizer; 15-30 drops to 2 ounces of lotion; 10-20 drops to 8 ounces of shampoo; 15-30 drops to 8 ounces of conditioner.

After Shower: After showering, while your skin is still wet, put 1-3 drops of essential oil in the palm of one of your hands and rub your hands together. Quickly and evenly spread the essential oil over your legs, arms, and torso. Avoid sensitive-skin areas. Wait for 30 seconds, breathing in the aroma, and then pat your skin dry.

Anointing Oil: Anointing oils are used for subtle aromatherapy and subtle energy work. Mix 1 drop of essential oil in 1 teaspoon of jojoba or olive oil.

Bath: Mix 4-8 drops of essential oil in 1 teaspoon of carrier oil, such as fractionated coconut oil. (You can also add the essential oil to ½ cup of whole milk or heavy cream.) Set aside. If you have muscle aches, add Epsom or Dead Sea salts. Fill the tub with warm water and immerse yourself. Add the essential oil mixture and swirl the water around you. Massage your skin and breathe in the aroma. Remain in the tub for 10-15 minutes.

Bath, Foot: Mix 1-3 drops of essential oil in ½ teaspoon of carrier oil, such as fractionated coconut oil. Set aside. Fill a tub (deep enough to cover your feet and ankles) with warm water. Add the essential oil mixture, stir well, and immerse your feet for 10-15 minutes. Breathe in the aroma and massage your feet.

Body Lotion: Add 6-30 drops of essential oil in 1 ounce of fragrance-free, natural moisturizing lotion. Apply to your skin, especially after a shower or bath.

Body Oil: Mix 6-30 drops of essential oil in 1 ounce of carrier, such as fractionated coconut oil or sweet almond oil. Apply to your skin, especially after a shower or bath.

Chest Rub: Mix 5-15 drops of essential oil in 1 tablespoon of carrier oil or fragrance-free, natural lotion. Apply to upper chest and upper back.

Compress: Fill a basin with water. (Warm water relaxes and increases circulation. Cool water invigorates and relieves inflammation.) Add 3-5 drops of essential oil and briskly stir. Lay in a washcloth, wring, and apply to the area in need. Dip, wring, and apply 3 more times. Leave the last compress in place for 3 minutes.

Compress, Facial: Fill the sink with warm water. Add 1-3 drops of essential oil in the water and agitate the water to mix well. Lay in a clean washcloth, wring, and apply to face, with eyes closed, holding in place for 5-10 seconds. Repeat dipping, wringing, and applying—3 times. Pat dry.

Diffusion: Follow diffuser manufacturer's instructions to fill the air with therapeutic aroma.

Facial Oil: Mix 2-5 drops of essential oil in 1 ounce of carrier such as jojoba, olive oil, or rose hip seed oil.

Inhalation: Put 1-3 drops of essential oil on a tissue and inhale the aroma through your nose. Pause and inhale again. (Avoid touching your nose with the tissue.)

Inhalation, Hot Water: Add 1-2 drops of essential oil in a small bowl of hot water. Keeping your eyes tightly closed, lean over the bowl and breathe in deeply yet gently and exhale. Continue for 30 seconds. Inhale through your nose for respiratory or sinus conditions, and through your mouth for throat issues or coughs. Repeat as desired.

Massage: Mix 6-30 drops of essential oil in 1 ounce of carrier oil or fragrance-free, natural lotion.

Perfume: Mix 10-20 drops of essential oil in 1 tablespoon of jojoba. Apply to pulse points, such as inner wrists, behind knees, or backs of ankles.

Room Mist: Mix 30-60 drops of essential oil in 4 ounces of water in a mister bottle. Shake well before each use and avoid getting it into the eyes.

Skin Mist: Mix 10-40 drops of essential oil in 4 ounces of water in a mister bottle. Shake well before each use and avoid getting it into the eyes.

Scalp Oil: Mix 12-24 drops of essential oil in 2 ounces of fractionated coconut oil or jojoba, or a blend of both. Store in a glass bottle with a cap. Use about 1 teaspoon to massage into scalp at night. Shampoo in the morning.

Spot Application: Mix 1-4 drops of essential oil in 1 teaspoon of carrier oil or aloe vera and apply to the specific area in need.

General Dilution Rates

1% dilution - 1 drop of essential oil per 5ml (100 drops) or 1 tsp of carrier oil
6 drops of essential oil per 1 oz of carrier oil

2% dilution - 2 drops of essential oil per 5ml (100 drops) or 1 tsp of carrier oil
12 drops of essential oil per 1 oz of carrier oil

3% dilution - 3 drops of essential oil per 5ml (100 drops) or 1 tsp of carrier oil
18 drops of essential oil per 1 oz of carrier oil

4% dilution - 4 drops of essential oil per 5ml (100 drops) or 1 tsp of carrier oil
24 drops of essential oil per 1 oz of carrier oil

5% dilution - 5 drops of essential oil per 5ml (100 drops) or 1 tsp of carrier oil
30 drops of essential oil per 1 oz of carrier oil

Quick Reference Guide

Adaptogenic: Has a balancing effect on physiological functions and mental states, increasing resistance to stress. *Lavender, Geranium, Rosewood*

Analgesic: Relieves pain. *German Chamomile, Roman Chamomile, Lavender, Eucalyptus Globulus, Eucalyptus Citriodora, Peppermint, Bay Laurel, Black Pepper, Geranium, Ginger, Nutmeg, Coriander, Rosemary, Clove Bud, Marjoram Sweet, Plai, Wintergreen, Niaouli*

Antiallergenic: Relieves or reduces symptoms of an allergic reaction. *German Chamomile, Blue Tansy, Helichrysum*

Antibacterial: Fights bacterial infections. *Tea Tree, Oregano, Thyme ct. linalol, Niaouli, Lavender, Eucalyptus Globulus, Eucalyptus Radiata, Eucalyptus Citriodora, Lemon, Peppermint, Myrrh, Clove Bud, Lemongrass, Plai*

Antidepressant: Uplifts the mind, counteracts melancholy, and promotes a positive attitude. *Bergamot, Clary Sage, Geranium, Grapefruit, Jasmine, Lavender, Lemon, Lemongrass, Orange, Petitgrain, Neroli, Rose, Rosemary, Ylang Ylang*

Antifungal: Fights fungal infections. *Geranium, Thyme ct. linalol, Tea Tree, Palmarosa, Patchouli, Lemongrass, Eucalyptus Citriodora, Clove Bud, Petitgrain, Cinnamon Leaf, Myrrh*

Anti-inflammatory: Relieves or reduces inflammation. *German Chamomile, Roman Chamomile, Helichrysum, Lavender, Rose, Tea Tree, Sandalwood, Plai, Niaouli, Blue Tansy, Petitgrain, Cardamom, Eucalyptus Radiata*

Antineuralgic: Relieves or reduces nerve pain. *Nutmeg, Lavender, German Chamomile, Roman Chamomile, Sandalwood, Clove Bud, Eucalyptus Globulus, Eucalyptus Radiata, Marjoram Sweet, Helichrysum, Black Pepper, Bay Laurel, Ginger, Peppermint, Coriander, Valerian Root*

Antipruritic: Relieves or reduces itching. *German Chamomile, Roman Chamomile, Peppermint, Spearmint, Lavender, Tea Tree, Lemon*

Antiseptic: Helps control infections and prevent tissue degeneration. (Most essential oils have some antiseptic properties.) *Lavender, Tea Tree, Niaouli, Thyme ct. linalol, Lemon, Geranium, German Chamomile, Roman Chamomile, Rose, Helichrysum, Eucalyptus Globulus, Eucalyptus Radiata, Eucalyptus Citriodora, Ravensara, Ravintsara, Bay Laurel, Marjoram Spanish, Palmarosa, Basil, Clary Sage, Clove Bud, Neroli, Cypress, Frankincense, Cedarwood, Juniper Berry, Lemongrass, Fir, Myrrh, Bergamot, Peppermint, Pine, Nutmeg, Ginger, Rosemary, Sandalwood, Rosewood, Oregano, Vetiver, Plai, Benzoin, Camphor White, Cinnamon, Sage, Yuzu*

Antispasmodic: Relieves or reduces muscle spasms and cramps. *German Chamomile, Roman Chamomile, Clary Sage, Lavender, Petitgrain, Marjoram Sweet, Sandalwood, Peppermint, Cardamom, Ginger, Black Pepper, Eucalyptus Globulus, Thyme ct. linalol, Basil, Helichrysum*

Antitussive: Reduces coughing by calming the coughing reflex. *Peppermint, Cypress, Black Spruce, Sandalwood*

Antiviral: Fights viral infections. *Eucalyptus Globulus, Eucalyptus Radiata, Tea Tree, Thyme ct. linalol, Niaouli, Bay Laurel, Ravintsara, Ravensara, Myrrh, Palmarosa, Cinnamon Leaf, Helichrysum, Lemongrass, Lemon, Clove Bud*

Aphrodisiac: Promotes sexual desire. *Cardamom, Clary Sage, Black Pepper, Ginger, Jasmine, Nutmeg, Patchouli, Rose, Sandalwood, Vetiver, Ylang Ylang*

Cicatrisant: Encourages rapid skin cell regeneration and wound healing. *Helichrysum, Lavender, Geranium, Frankincense, German Chamomile, Roman Chamomile, Rose, Cypress, Eucalyptus Globulus, Neroli, Juniper Berry, Lemon, Niaouli, Patchouli, Tea Tree, Myrrh*

Decongestant: Clears respiratory congestion. *Eucalyptus Globulus, Eucalyptus Radiata, Rosemary, Spike Lavender, Bay Laurel, Peppermint, Pine, Eucalyptus Smithii, Fir Balsam, Fir Douglas, Spearmint*

Deodorant: Corrects, masks, or improves unpleasant odors. *Bergamot, Clary Sage, Coriander, Cypress, Eucalyptus Globulus, Eucalyptus Radiata, Eucalyptus Citriodora, Geranium, Lavender, Lemongrass, Lemon, Peppermint, Patchouli, Pine, Thyme ct. linalol, Rosewood, Petitgrain, Yuzu*

Euphoric: Promotes a sense of happiness and well-being. *Clary Sage, Ylang Ylang, Jasmine*

Immune Support: Supports the immune response. *Tea Tree, Lavender, Frankincense, Bay Laurel, Ravensara, Ravintsara, Eucalyptus Globulus, Eucalyptus Radiata, Niaouli, Geranium, Helichrysum, Palmarosa, Thyme ct. linalol, Bergamot, Lemon, Vetiver*

Nervine: Supports and benefits the nervous system. Calming nervines (*) can reduce stress and anxiety. Stimulating nervines (#) can revive and rejuvenate. *Roman Chamomile*, Clary Sage*, Ylang Ylang*, Lavender*, Marjoram Sweet*, Sandalwood*, Vetiver*, Basil#, Rosemary#, Peppermint#, Juniper Berry#*

Restorative: Strengthens and revives the body or parts of the body. *Rosemary, Black Spruce, Pine, Basil, Lime, Spearmint*

Rubefacient: Increases/stimulates local circulation and warms. *Black Pepper, Ginger, Rosemary, Eucalyptus Globulus, Bay Laurel, Juniper Berry*

Sedative: Relaxes, calms, or reduces a physiological function. *Roman Chamomile, Clary Sage, Frankincense, Jasmine, Lavender, Marjoram Sweet, Neroli, Rose, Bergamot, Sandalwood, Vetiver, Ylang Ylang, Benzoin*

Stimulant: Stimulates or quickens a physiological function. *Black Pepper, Rosemary, Cardamom, Eucalyptus Globulus, Nutmeg, Ginger, Pine, Bay Laurel, Peppermint, Juniper Berry, Tea Tree, Camphor White, Cinnamon, Spearmint*

Key Essential Oils for Systems of the Body

Circulatory (blood and lymph):

Rosemary, Black Pepper, Marjoram Sweet, Juniper Berry, Geranium, Eucalyptus Globulus

Digestive:

Peppermint, Cardamom, Ginger, Basil, Fennel

Endocrine:

Lavender, Geranium, Tea Tree, Frankincense

Immune:

Tea Tree, Lavender, Frankincense, Bay Laurel, Ravintsara, Eucalyptus Globulus, Eucalyptus Radiata, Niaouli

Integumentary (skin):

Lavender, Frankincense, Geranium, Neroli, Rose, Sandalwood, German Chamomile, Ylang Ylang, Carrot Seed

Musculoskeletal:

Lavender, Rosemary, Black Pepper, Marjoram Sweet, German Chamomile

Nervous:

To calm – Roman Chamomile, Clary Sage, Ylang Ylang, Lavender, Sandalwood, Bergamot

To stimulate – Rosemary, Peppermint, Juniper Berry

Reproductive:

Female – Geranium, Lavender, Rose, Clary Sage, Frankincense

Male – Pine, Tea Tree, Lavender

Respiratory:

Eucalyptus Globulus, Eucalyptus Radiata, Lavender, Tea Tree, Rosemary, Sandalwood

Urinary:

Lavender, Geranium, Tea Tree

Essential Oil Testing

Essential 3 uses the following methods to test their essential oils to insure therapeutic quality for their customers.

- **GC/GLC:** Gas Chromatography or Gas Liquid Chromatography. GC/GLC is a measurement tool that vaporizes each molecule of the essential oil and quantifies the percentage of the constituent present. It does not identify the constituent.

- **MS:** Mass Spectrometry. MS determines the molecular mass of each molecule of the essential oil and identifies each constituent.

- **FID:** Flame Ionization Detection (used in conjunction with gas chromatography). FID provides increased accuracy in the quantitative results specific to GC test information.

References and Recommended Reading

*The Aromatherapy Practitioner
Reference Manual*
by Sylla Shepard-Hangar

The Directory of Essential Oils
by Wanda Sellar

Practical Aromatherapy For Self Care
by Joni Keim

Holistic Aromatherapy for Animals
by Kristen Leigh Bell

Advanced Aromatherapy
by Dr. Kurt Schnaubelt

Aromatherapy & Subtle Energy Techniques
by Joni Keim & Ruah Bull

Daily Aromatherapy
by Joni Keim & Ruah Bull

Aromatherapy Anointing Oils
by Joni Keim & Ruah Bull

Clinical Aromatherapy
by Jane Buckle

Aromatherapy for Massage Practitioners
by Ingrid Martin

Essential Chemistry for Safe Aromatherapy
by Sue Clarke

Clinical Aromatherapy for Pregnancy and Childbirth
by Denise Tiran

Aromatherapy for the Healthy Child
by Valerie Ann Worwood

Aromatherapy: A Complete Guide to the Healing Art
by Kathi Keville & Mindy Green   (Second Edition)

Scents and Scentuality
by Valerie Ann Worwood

The Fragrant Mind
by Valerie Ann Worwood

Aromatherapy for Health Professionals
by Shirley Price & Len Price

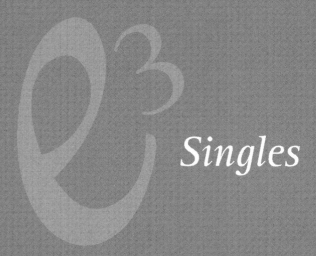

Singles

100% PURE THERAPEUTIC-QUALITY ESSENTIAL OILS

"Look in the perfume of flowers and of nature
for peace of mind and joy of life."
                    — Wang Wei, 8th century

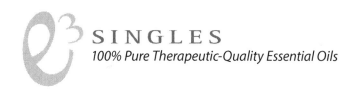

SINGLES
100% Pure Therapeutic-Quality Essential Oils

Basil, ct. linalol

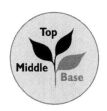

Latin name: *Ocimum basilicum*

Country of origin: USA

Part of the plant: Leaves and flowering tops

Extraction method: Steam distilled

Main biochemical components*: Linalol, 1,8 cineole, para-cymene

Physical uses: Indigestion, nausea, stomach spasms, menstrual cramps, muscle strain, stiff joints, infections, respiratory congestion, poor circulation, nervous tension.

Skin care uses: Skin tonic, insect bites, infections, scalp tonic, insect repellant.

Psychological uses: Nervous tension, insomnia, mild depression, stress, anxiety, mental fog, mental fatigue.

Subtle uses: Clears and uplifts the mind. Promotes intuition.

Notes: Use Basil, ct. linalol in a 1-5% dilution. Avoid during pregnancy and nursing.

*Chemical component percentages may vary. Essential 3 offers a *Certificate of Analysis* for review.

Methods of use:

After Shower	Chest Rub
Compress	Diffusion
Inhalation	Massage
Anointing Oil	Scalp Oil
Spot Application	

For more information, see Methods of Using Essential Oils on page xi.

NOTES

Avoid during pregnancy and nursing

Digestive tonic

Which One?

Basil, ct. linalol has a soft, warm aroma. Its action is balancing & toning. Basil, ct. methyl chavicol has a warm, peppery aroma. Its action is more stimulating. Their uses are somewhat interchangeable—both being good for cramps, immune support, and mental alertness.

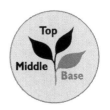

Top
Middle
Base

NOTES

Avoid during pregnancy
Outstanding for
menstrual cramps
Poison oak relief

Basil, ct. methyl chavicol

Latin name: *Ocimum basilicum*

Country of origin: USA

Part of the plant: Leaves and flowering tops

Extraction method: Steam distilled

Main biochemical components*: Methyl chavicol, linalol, limonene

Physical uses: Muscle aches, muscle strain, muscle spasms such as menstrual and stomach cramps, indigestion, nausea, stiff joints, infections, respiratory congestion, coughs, nervous tension.

Skin care uses: Skin tonic, insect bites, infections, scalp tonic, insect repellant.

Psychological uses: Nervous tension, insomnia, mild depression, stress, anxiety, mental fog, mental fatigue.

Subtle uses: Clears and uplifts the mind. Promotes intuition.

Notes: Use Basil, ct. methyl chavicol in a 1-5% dilution.
Avoid during pregnancy and nursing.

* Chemical component percentages may vary.
Essential 3 offers a *Certificate of Analysis* for review.

Methods of use:

After Shower	Chest Rub
Compress	Diffusion
Inhalation	Massage
Anointing Oil	Scalp Oil
Spot Application	

For more information, see Methods of Using Essential Oils on page xi.

Which One?

Basil, ct. linalol has a soft, warm aroma. Its action is balancing & toning. **Basil, ct. methyl chavicol** has a warm, peppery aroma. Its action is more stimulating. Their uses are somewhat interchangeable—both being good for cramps, immune support, and mental alertness.

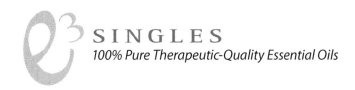

SINGLES
100% Pure Therapeutic-Quality Essential Oils

Bay Laurel

Latin name: *Laurus nobilis*

Country of origin: Crete

Part of the plant: Dried leaves

Extraction method: Steam distilled

Main biochemical components*: 1,8 cineole, linalol, alpha-terpinyl acetate

Physical uses: Respiratory congestion, muscle aches, stiff joints, poor circulation, headaches, infections, lymphatic support, immune support.

Skin care uses: Scalp tonic, blemishes, infections, bruises.

Psychological uses: Mental fatigue, mental fog, anxiety, fear.

Subtle uses: Promotes intuition. Clears mental blocks. Promotes confidence and courage.

Notes: Use Bay Laurel in a 1-5% dilution. Avoid during pregnancy and nursing.

* Chemical component percentages may vary. Essential 3 offers a *Certificate of Analysis* for review.

Methods of use:

After Shower	Chest Rub
Compress	Diffusion
Inhalation	Massage
Anointing Oil	Scalp Oil
Spot Application	

For more information, see Methods of Using Essential Oils on page xi.

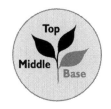

NOTES

Avoid during pregnancy and nursing

Immune Stimulant

Lymphatic Decongestant

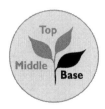

NOTES

May be sensitizing

Euphoric

Comforting

Vanilla-like aroma

Benzoin

Latin name: *Styrax benzoin*

Country of origin: Laos

Part of the plant: Resin

Extraction method: Absolute

Main biochemical components*: Benzoic acid, coniferyl benzoate

Physical uses: Body chills, stiff joints, infections, coughs, colds, flu, irritated throats.

Skin care uses: Irritations, itches, bruises, minor burns, small wounds, infections.

Psychological uses: Stress, nervous tension, emotional weakness, emotional coolness, mild depression.

Subtle uses: Grounds and comforts. Dispels anger and negativity. Focuses the mind for meditation and prayer.

Notes: Use Benzoin in a 1-5% dilution. May be sensitizing.

* Chemical component percentages may vary. Essential 3 offers a *Certificate of Analysis* for review.

Methods of use:

Body Lotion	Body Oil
Chest Rub	Inhalation, Hot Water
Inhalation	Massage
Annointing Oil	Spot Application

For more information, see Methods of Using Essential Oils on page xi.

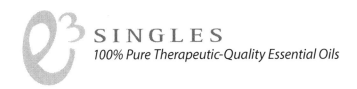

Bergamot

Latin name: *Citrus bergamia*

Country of origin: Italy

Part of the plant: Rinds

Extraction method: Cold pressed

Main biochemical components*: Linalyl acetate, limonene, linalol

Physical uses: Colds, flu, fevers, infections, immune support.

Skin care uses: Cold sores, oily skin, infections, small wounds, eczema, body odor.

Psychological uses: Mild depression, stress, anxiety, nervousness, mood swings, apathy.

Subtle uses: Brings in positive energy. Eases grief. Promotes self-love. Opens the heart.

Notes: Do not use Bergamot directly on the skin when you are going to be in the sun.

* Chemical component percentages may vary. Essential 3 offers a *Certificate of Analysis* for review.

Methods of use:

Bath	Bath, Foot
Chest Rub	Diffusion
Inhalation	Room Mist
Spot Application	Anointing Oil

For more information, see Methods of Using Essential Oils on page xi.

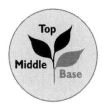

NOTES

Avoid use in sun

Stress relief

Anti-depressant

Hospice use for calming

Maybe more calming for some people than Lavender

Unique, appealing citrus aroma

Which One?
Bergamot has a fresh, bright, faintly floral, citrus aroma. It contains the naturally-occurring furocoumarins. Bergamot FCF has a slightly softer aroma. It has had the naturally-occurring furocoumarins removed. Their uses are interchangeable with the exception that Bergamot should not be used in the sun and Bergamot FCF is a safer choice to use in leave-on products .

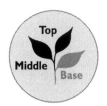

NOTES

Stress relief

Anti-depressant

Hospice use for calming

May be more calming
for some people than
Lavender

Which One?
Bergamot has a fresh, bright, faintly floral, citrus aroma. It contains the naturally-occurring furocoumarins. Bergamot FCF has a slightly softer aroma. It has had the naturally-occurring furocoumarins removed. Their uses are interchangeable with the exception that Bergamot should not be used in the sun and Bergamot FCF is a safer choice to use in leave-on products.

Bergamot, FCF

Latin name: *Citrus bergamia*

Country of origin: China

Part of the plant: Rinds

Extraction method: Cold pressed

Main biochemical components*: Limonene, linalyl acetate, linalol

Physical uses: Colds, flu, fevers, infections, immune support.

Skin care uses: Cold sores, oily skin, infections, small wounds, eczema, body odor.

Psychological uses: Mild depression, stress, anxiety, nervousness, mood swings, apathy.

Subtle uses: Brings in positive energy. Eases grief. Promotes self-love. Opens the heart.

Notes: FCF stands for furocoumarin-free. This form of Bergamot does not carry the concern for use in the sun, and can be used in products that are left on the skin.

* Chemical component percentages may vary. Essential 3 offers a *Certificate of Analysis* for review.

Methods of use:

After Shower	Bath
Bath, Foot	Body Lotion
Body Oil	Chest Rub
Compress	Diffusion
Inhalation	Massage
Room Mist	Spot Application
Anointing Oil	

For more information, see Methods of Using Essential Oils on page xi.

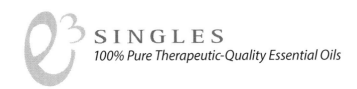

Black Pepper

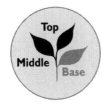

Latin name: *Piper nigrum*

Country of origin: India

Part of the plant: Dried, crushed fruit

Extraction method: Steam distilled

Main biochemical components*:
Beta-caryophyllene, limonene, sabinene

Physical uses: Muscle aches, stiff joints, poor circulation, feeling cold, indigestion, sluggish digestion, infections.

Skin care uses: n/a

Psychological uses: Mental fatigue or apathy.

Subtle uses: Dispels apathy.

Notes: Use Black Pepper in a 1-5% dilution.

* Chemical component percentages may vary. Essential 3 offers a *Certificate of Analysis* for review.

Methods of use:
Inhalation
Massage (specific area)
Spot Application
Anointing Oil

For more information, see Methods of Using Essential Oils on page xi.

NOTES

Stimulant

Warms muscles for

massage

Smoking cessation support

Chronic inflammation

from fibromyalgia

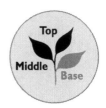

NOTES

May be sensitizing

*Avoid during pregnancy
and nursing*

Superior adrenal support

Respiratory tonic

Black Spruce

Latin name: *Picea mariana*

Country of origin: Canada

Part of the plant: Needles

Extraction method: Steam distilled

Main biochemical components*: Borynl acetate, camphene, pinene

Physical uses: Fatigue (especially after an illness), tired muscles, muscle aches, poor circulation, stiff joints, infections, respiratory congestion, immune support, adrenal support.

Skin care uses: Blemishes, infections, dry eczema.

Psychological uses: Stress, anxiety, burn out, mental fog.

Subtle uses: Clears and cleanses. Promotes intuition. Promotes mental clarity and objectivity.

Notes: Use Black Spruce in a 1-5% dilution. May be sensitizing. Avoid during pregnancy and nursing.

* Chemical component percentages may vary.
  Essential 3 offers a *Certificate of Analysis* for review.

Methods of use:

After Shower	Chest Rub
Compress	Diffusion
Inhalation	Massage
Room Mist	Spot Application
Anointing Oil	

For more information, see Methods of Using Essential Oils on page xi.

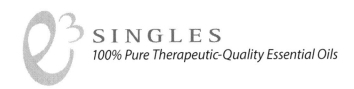
Camphor, White

Latin name: *Cinnamomum camphora*

Country of origin: China

Part of the plant: Wood, roots, branches

Extraction method: Steam distilled

Main biochemical components*: Camphor, safrole, 1,8 cineole

Physical uses: Respiratory congestion, colds, flu, coughs, muscle aches, inflammation, stiff joints, infections.

Skin care uses: Blemishes, oily skin, infections, insect repellant.

Psychological uses: Mental fatigue.

Subtle uses: Clears and cleanses. Strengthens.

Notes: Use Camphor in a 1-5% dilution. Avoid during pregnancy and nursing.

* Chemical component percentages may vary. Essential 3 offers a *Certificate of Analysis* for review.

Methods of use:

Chest Rub	Compress
Inhalation	Massage (specific area)
Spot Application	Anointing Oil

For more information, see Methods of Using Essential Oils on page xi.

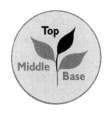

NOTES

Avoid during pregnancy and nursing

Stimulant

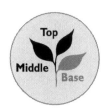

NOTES

Aphrodisiac

Air freshener

Cardamom

Latin name: *Elettaria cardamomum*

Country of origin: India

Part of the plant: Seeds of the dried, ripe fruit

Extraction method: Steam distilled

Main biochemical components*: Alpha-terpinyl acetate, 1,8 cineole, linalyl acetate

Physical uses: Indigestion, nausea, heartburn, stomach ache, poor circulation, feeling cold, muscle spasms, respiratory congestion, coughs.

Skin care uses: n/a

Psychological uses: Anxiety, mental fatigue, mild depression, low libido, emotional coolness.

Subtle uses: Promotes enthusiasm.

Notes: Use Cardamom in a 1-5% dilution.

* Chemical component percentages may vary.
    Essential 3 offers a *Certificate of Analysis* for review.

Methods of use:

Chest Rub	Compress
Diffusion	Inhalation
Massage	Spot Application
Anointing Oil	

For more information, see Methods of Using Essential Oils on page xi.

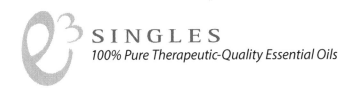

SINGLES
100% Pure Therapeutic-Quality Essential Oils

Carrot Seed

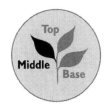

Latin name: *Daucus carota*

Country of origin: France

Part of the plant: Seeds

Extraction method: Steam distilled

Main biochemical components*: Carotol, geranyl acetate, alpha-pinene

Physical uses: Indigestion, lymphatic support, liver tonic, digestive tonic.

Skin care uses: Dry skin, sun-damaged skin, mature skin, devitalized skin, eczema, scars, calluses, rashes, burns, couperose, rosacea, skin tonic.

Psychological uses: Anxiety, stress, exhaustion.

Subtle uses: Clears energy blocks.

Notes: Avoid Carrot Seed during pregnancy and nursing.

* Chemical component percentages may vary. Essential 3 offers a *Certificate of Analysis* for review.

Methods of use:

Add to Products	After Shower
Bath	Bath, Foot
Body Lotion	Body Oil
Compress	Compress, Facial
Facial Oil	Inhalation
Massage	Skin Mist
Spot Application	Anointing Oil

For more information, see Methods of Using Essential Oils on page xi.

NOTES

Avoid during pregnancy and nursing

Liver support

Skin care

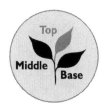

NOTES

Avoid during pregnancy
and nursing
Meditation

Cedarwood, Atlas

Latin name: *Cedrus atlantica*

Country of origin: Morocco

Part of the plant: Wood

Extraction method: Steam distilled

Main biochemical components*:
Beta-himachalene, alpha-himachalene, gamma-himachalene

Physical uses: Muscle aches, stiff joints, poor lymphatic circulation, respiratory congestion, bronchitis, coughs, infections, water retention, immune support.

Skin care uses: Oily skin, dermatitis, blemishes, infections, dandruff, scalp tonic.

Psychological uses: Stress, tension, anxiety, emotional exhaustion, emotional instability.

Subtle uses: Clears and cleanses. Brings in positive energy. Strengthens confidence and will. Steadies the mind and promotes a meditative state.

Notes: Use Cedarwood, Atlas in a 1-5% dilution. Avoid during pregnancy and nursing.

* Chemical component percentages may vary.
  Essential 3 offers a *Certificate of Analysis* for review.

Methods of use:

Bath	Bath, Foot
Chest Rub	Compress
Diffusion	Inhalation
Inhalation, Hot Water	Massage
Scalp Oil	Spot Application
Anointing Oil	

For more information, see Methods of Using Essential Oils on page xi.

Which One?

Cedarwood, Atlas has a soft, woody, sweet, warm aroma. **Cedarwood (USA)** has a rich, dry, woody, balsamic aroma, and is part of the juniper family. It is not a true cedar. Their uses are generally interchangeable—both being good for lymphatic support, respiratory congestion, and stress.

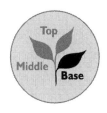

Cedarwood (USA)

Latin name: *Juniperus virginiana*

Country of origin: USA

Part of the plant: Wood

Extraction method: Steam distilled

Main biochemical components*: Sesquiterpene hydrocarbons, cedrol, sesquiterpenes

Physical uses: Muscle aches, muscle spasms, stiff joints, poor circulation, respiratory congestion, bronchitis, sinusitis, coughs, infections, lymphatic support.

Skin care uses: Oily skin, dermatitis, blemishes, dandruff, scalp tonic, infections, insect repellant.

Psychological uses: Stress, tension, anxiety, emotional instability.

Subtle uses: Clears and cleanses. Brings in positive energy. Strengthens confidence and will.

Notes: Use Cedarwood (USA) in a 1-5% dilution. May be sensitizing. Avoid during pregnancy and nursing.

* Chemical component percentages may vary. Essential 3 offers a *Certificate of Analysis* for review.

Methods of use:

Bath	Bath, Foot
Chest Rub	Compress
Diffusion	Inhalation
Inhalation, Hot Water	Massage
Scalp Oil	Spot Application
Anointing Oil	

For more information, see Methods of Using Essential Oils on page xi.

NOTES

May be sensitizing

Avoid during pregnancy and nursing

Moth repellant (refresh cedar blocks)

Which One?

Cedarwood, Atlas has a soft, woody, sweet, warm aroma. **Cedarwood (USA)** has a rich, dry, woody, balsamic aroma, and is part of the juniper family. It is not a true cedar. Their uses are generally interchangeable—both being good for lymphatic support, respiratory congestion, and stress.

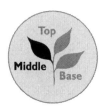

NOTES

Unsurpassed

anti-inflammatory

Skin care

Sleep aid

Stress relief

Chamomile, German

Latin name: *Matricaria chamomilla*

Country of origin: Bulgaria

Part of the plant: Flowers

Extraction method: Steam distilled

Main biochemical components*: Chamazulene, bisabolol oxide, bisabolone oxide

Physical uses: Inflamed muscles and joints, infections, headaches, indigestion, nerve pain.

Skin care uses: Inflammation, irritations, rashes, allergic reactions, acne, rosacea, sunburn, itching, small cuts, minor burns, infections, insect bites and stings.

Psychological uses: Stress, tension, anxiety, anger, fear, sleeplessness, impatience.

Subtle uses: Calms. Supports calm, truthful communication.

Notes: Chamomile, German is one of the best essential oils for inflammation.

* Chemical component percentages may vary. Essential 3 offers a *Certificate of Analysis* for review.

Methods of use:

Add to Products	After Shower
Bath	Bath, Foot
Body Lotion	Body Oil
Compress	Compress, Facial
Diffusion	Facial Oil
Inhalation	Massage
Skin Mist	Spot Application
Anointing Oil	

For more information, see Methods of Using Essential Oils on page xi.

Which One?

Chamomile, German has a sweet, warm, herbaceous aroma. Chamomile, Roman has a fresh, sweet, apple-like aroma. They are both good for skin care. Choose **German** for inflammation or allergic reactions. Choose **Roman** for aches, cramps, and nervous system issues.

Chamomile, Roman

Latin name: *Anthemis nobilis*

Country of origin: USA

Part of the plant: Flowering tops

Extraction method: Steam distilled

Main biochemical components*: Isoamyl angelate, isobutyl angelate, 2-methylbutyl 2-methylbutyrate

Physical uses: Muscle aches, muscle spasms and cramps, stiff joints, menstrual cramps, headaches, inflammation, chronic infections, stomach ache, PMS, nerve pain.

Skin care uses: Inflammation, irritations, rashes, allergic reactions, acne, rosacea, sunburn, itching, minor burns, small cuts, chronic infections, insect bites and stings.

Psychological uses: Stress, tension, anxiety, anger, fear, sleeplessness, worry, shock, impatience.

Subtle uses: Calms. Promotes patience. Eases grief and sadness.

Notes: Avoid Chamomile, Roman during the first 4 months of pregnancy.

* Chemical component percentages may vary. Essential 3 offers a *Certificate of Analysis* for review.

Methods of use:

Add to Products	After Shower
Bath	Bath, Foot
Body Lotion	Body Oil
Compress	Compress, Facial
Diffusion	Facial Oil
Inhalation	Massage
Room Mist	Skin Mist
Spot Application	Anointing Oil

For more information, see Methods of Using Essential Oils on page xi.

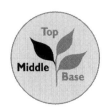

NOTES

Avoid during the first 4 months of pregnancy

Stress relief

Skin care

Menstrual cramps (especially with Basil ct. methyl chavicol)

To calm before surgery (a drop on hospital gown)

Sleep aid

Which One?

Chamomile, German has a sweet, warm, herbaceous aroma. **Chamomile, Roman** has a fresh, sweet, apple-like aroma. They are both good for skin care. Choose **German** for inflammation or allergic reactions. Choose **Roman** for aches, cramps, and nervous system issues.

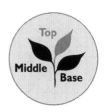

Top
Middle
Base

NOTES

Use highly diluted!

(1% or less)

May be sensitizing

Avoid during pregnancy

and nursing

Highly anti-infectious

Cinnamon Leaf

Latin name: *Cinnamomum zeylanicum*

Country of origin: Sri Lanka

Part of the plant: Leaves

Extraction method: Steam distilled

Main biochemical components*: Eugenol, (E)-cinnamic aldehyde, benzyl benzoate

Physical uses: Infections (viral, bacterial, fungal), bronchitis, colds, flu, poor circulation, immune support.

Skin care uses: Warts, head lice, infections (viral, bacterial, fungal).

Psychological uses: Exhaustion, mild depression, emotional coolness, low libido.

Subtle uses: Strengthens intuition. Promotes creativity.

Notes: Use Cinnamon Leaf highly diluted (1% or less)! May be sensitizing. Avoid during pregnancy and nursing.

* Chemical component percentages may vary. Essential 3 offers a *Certificate of Analysis* for review.

Methods of use:

Chest Rub	Inhalation
Massage	Spot Application
Anointing Oil	

For more information, see Methods of Using Essential Oils on page xi.

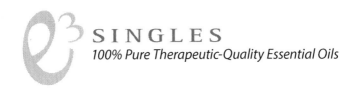
Citronella

Latin name: *Cymbopogon winterianus*

Country of origin: Indonesia

Part of the plant: Grass

Extraction method: Steam distilled

Main biochemical components*: Citronellal, geraniol, citronellol

Physical uses: Stiff joints, inflammation, colds, flu, infections. Insect repellant.

Skin care uses: n/a

Psychological uses: Mental fatigue, stress, anxiety.

Subtle uses: Balances the first through fifth energy centers. Calms anger.

Notes: Use Citronella in a 1-5% dilution. May be sensitizing.

* Chemical component percentages may vary. Essential 3 offers a *Certificate of Analysis* for review.

Methods of use:

Diffusion	Inhalation
Massage	Room Mist
Spot Application	Anointing Oil

For more information, see Methods of Using Essential Oils on page xi.

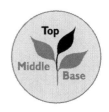

NOTES

May be sensitizing

Insect repellant

Bright, lemony aroma

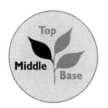

N O T E S

Avoid during pregnancy
and nursing

Euphoric

PMS

Menopause

Clary Sage

Latin name: *Salvia sclarea*

Country of origin: USA

Part of the plant: Flowering tops

Extraction method: Steam distilled

Main biochemical components*: Linalyl acetate, linalol, germacrene-D

Physical uses: Muscle aches, spasms, and cramps, PMS, menopausal symptoms, poor circulation, poor digestion, infections.

Skin care uses: Oily skin, blemishes, infections, dandruff.

Psychological uses: Stress, tension, anxiety, lack of sense of well-being, mild depression, fear, panic.

Subtle uses: Calms the energy centers. Inspires. Strengthens inner vision.

Notes: Avoid Clary Sage during pregnancy and nursing.

* Chemical component percentages may vary.
   Essential 3 offers a *Certificate of Analysis* for review.

Methods of use:

Add to Products	After Shower
Bath	Bath, Foot
Body Lotion	Body Oil
Compress	Compress, Facial
Diffusion	Facial Oil
Inhalation	Massage
Room Mist	Skin Mist
Scalp Oil	Spot Application
Anointing Oil	

For more information, see Methods of Using Essential Oils on page xi.

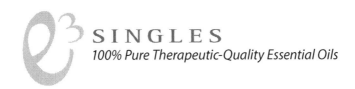

Clove Bud

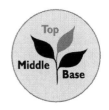

Latin name: *Eugenia caryophyllata*

Country of origin: Indonesia

Part of the plant: Dried buds

Extraction method: Steam distilled

Main biochemical components*: Eugenol, eugenyl acetate, caryophyllene

Physical uses: Muscle aches, stiff joints, infections, colds, flu, sinusitis, bronchitis, nausea, poor digestion, poor circulation.

Skin care uses: Athlete's foot, bruises, warts, blemishes, infections.

Psychological uses: Mental fatigue, mild depression, low libido.

Subtle uses: Promotes courage. Strengthens the conscious mind.

Notes: Use Clove Bud in a 1-5% dilution. May be sensitizing.

* Chemical component percentages may vary. Essential 3 offers a *Certificate of Analysis* for review.

Methods of use:

Chest Rub	Inhalation
Massage (specific area)	Spot Application
Anointing Oil	

For more information, see Methods of Using Essential Oils on page xi.

NOTES

May be sensitizing

Highly anti-infectious

Gum/dental pain relief

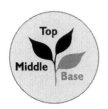

Top
Middle
Base

NOTES

Avoid during pregnancy and nursing.

Gentle, mental stimulant

Aphrodisiac

Coriander

Latin name: *Coriandrum sativum*

Country of origin: USA

Part of the plant: Dried, crushed seeds

Extraction method: Steam distilled

Main biochemical components*: Linalol, camphor, gamma-terpinene

Physical uses: Nausea, indigestion, upset stomach, infections, muscle aches, tight muscles, joint stiffness, nerve pain.

Skin care uses: n/a

Psychological uses: Nervous tension, nervous exhaustion, mental fatigue, low libido.

Subtle uses: Promotes confidence, creativity, spontaneity, and passion.

Notes: Use Coriander in a 1-5% dilution. Avoid during pregnancy and nursing.

* Chemical component percentages may vary. Essential 3 offers a *Certificate of Analysis* for review.

Methods of use:

Bath	Bath, Foot
Compress	Diffusion
Inhalation	Massage
Room Mist	Spot Application
Anointing Oil	

For more information, see Methods of Using Essential Oils on page xi.

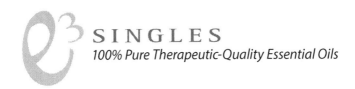
Cypress

Latin name: *Cupressus sempervirens*

Country of origin: Crete

Part of the plant: Needles and twigs

Extraction method: Steam distilled

Main biochemical components*: Alpha-pinene, delta-3-carene, cedrol

Physical uses: Throat and sinus infections, poor circulation, muscle aches, muscle cramps and spasms, water retention, PMS, menopausal symptoms, lymphatic support.

Skin care uses: Oily skin, blemishes, infections, poor circulation, excessive perspiration, body odor, small wounds.

Psychological uses: Nervous tension, mental fog.

Subtle uses: Strengthens and comforts, especially in times of change. Promotes confidence, patience, and wisdom. Clears energy blocks.

Notes: Avoid Cypress with high blood pressure. Avoid during pregnancy and nursing.

* Chemical component percentages may vary. Essential 3 offers a *Certificate of Analysis* for review.

Methods of use:

After Shower	Bath
Bath, Foot	Chest Rub
Compress	Diffusion
Facial Oil	Inhalation
Inhalation, Hot Water	Massage
Room Mist	Skin Mist
Spot Application	Anointing Oil

For more information, see Methods of Using Essential Oils on page xi.

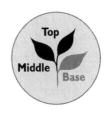

NOTES

Avoid w/ high blood

pressure

Avoid during

pregnancy

and nursing

Lymphatic

decongestant

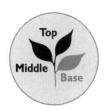

NOTES

A relaxing Eucalyptus

Insect repellant

Air freshener (especially
for sick rooms)

Eucalyptus, Citriodora

Latin name: *Eucalyptus citriodora*

Country of origin: China

Part of the plant: Leaves

Extraction method: Steam distilled

Main biochemical components*: Citronellal, isoisopulegol, 1, 8 cineole

Physical uses: Muscle aches, joint stiffness, sore throats, inflammation, colds, flu, infections, immune support, recuperation from long illness.

Skin care uses: Dandruff, athlete's foot, infections,

Psychological uses: Nervous tension, stress, anxiety, mild depression.

Subtle uses: Clears and balances the energy centers.

Notes: Eucalyptus, Citriodora is a unique Eucalyptus with relaxing qualities.

* Chemical component percentages may vary.
    Essential 3 offers a *Certificate of Analysis* for review.

Methods of use:

After Shower	Bath, Foot
Chest Rub	Compress
Diffusion	Inhalation
Scalp Oil	Inhalation, Hot Water
Massage	Room Mist
Spot Application	Anointing Oil

For more information, see Methods of Using Essential Oils on page xi.

Which One?

As a whole, the Eucalyptuses are for respiratory congestion and infection, immune support, and muscle aches. Their aromas are strong, refreshing, and camphoraceous. All are more or less stimulating except **Euc. Citriodora.** Choose **Euc. Globulus** for its strength, **Euc. Radiata** for longer-term use and its pleasant aroma, **Euc. Citriodora** for air disinfecting and night-time use, and **Euc. Smithii** for prevention, muscle and joint aches, and its mildness.

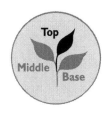

Eucalyptus, Globulus

Latin name: *Eucalyptus globulus*

Country of origin: Australia

Part of the plant: Leaves

Extraction method: Steam distilled

Main biochemical components*: 1,8 cineole, pinene, globulol

Physical uses: Respiratory congestion, colds, flu, sinusitis, bronchitis, sore throats, infections (viral, bacterial, fungal), fevers, muscle aches, stiff joints, poor circulation, headaches, immune support.

Skin care uses: Infections (viral, bacterial, fungal), insect bites, cold sores, devitalized skin condition.

Psychological uses: Mental fatigue, mental fog.

Subtle uses: Clears energy blocks. Inspires.

Notes: Avoid Eucalyptus, Globulus with high blood pressure. Avoid during pregnancy and nursing.

* Chemical component percentages may vary. Essential 3 offers a *Certificate of Analysis* for review.

NOTES

Avoid w/high blood pressure

Avoid during pregnancy and nursing

Immune stimulant

Spa towels (1 drop in water that moistens towels)

Exceptionally penetrating

May not be compatible with homeopathics

Methods of use:

After Shower	Bath
Bath, Foot	Chest Rub
Compress	Diffusion
Inhalation	Inhalation, Hot Water
Massage	Room Mist
Spot Application	Anointing Oil

For more information, see Methods of Using Essential Oils on page xi.

Which One?

As a whole, the Eucalyptuses are for respiratory congestion and infection, immune support, and muscle aches. Their aromas are strong, refreshing, and camphoraceous. All are more or less stimulating except **Euc. Citriodora.** Choose **Euc. Globulus** for its strength, **Euc. Radiata** for longer-term use and its pleasant aroma, **Euc. Citriodora** for air disinfecting and night-time use, and **Euc. Smithii** for prevention, muscle and joint aches, and its mildness.

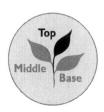

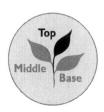

SINGLES
100% Pure Therapeutic-Quality Essential Oils

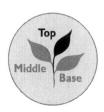

NOTES

Avoid during pregnancy

and nursing

Suited for long-term use

Steam room

A drop on tissue in

pillowcase for sinus issues

May not be compatible

with homeopathics

Eucalyptus, Radiata

Latin name: *Eucalyptus radiata*

Country of origin: Australia

Part of the plant: Leaves

Extraction method: Steam distilled

Main biochemical components*: 1,8 cineole, alpha-terpineol, alpha-terpinyl acetate

Physical uses: Respiratory congestion, colds, flu, sinusitis, bronchitis, sore throats, infections (viral, bacterial), fevers, muscle aches, stiff joints, inflammation, headaches, immune support.

Skin care uses: Infections (viral, bacterial), insect bites, cold sores, devitalized skin condition.

Psychological uses: Mild depression, apathy.

Subtle uses: Clears energy blocks. Inspires.

Notes: Avoid Eucalyptus, Radiata during pregnancy and nursing.

* Chemical component percentages may vary.
   Essential 3 offers a *Certificate of Analysis* for review.

Methods of use:

After Shower	Bath
Bath, Foot	Chest Rub
Compress	Diffusion
Inhalation	Inhalation, Hot Water
Massage	Room Mist
Spot Application	Anointing Oil

For more information, see Methods of Using Essential Oils on page xi.

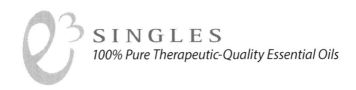
Eucalyptus, Smithii

Latin name: *Eucalyptus smithii*

Country of origin: Australia

Part of the plant: Leaves

Extraction method: Steam distilled

Main biochemical components*: 1,8 cineole, pinene, limonene

Physical uses: Respiratory congestion, colds, flu, sinusitis, bronchitis, sore throats, infections (viral, bacterial), muscle aches, stiff joints, inflammation, headaches, immune support.

Skin care uses: Infections (viral, bacterial), insect bites, cold sores, devitalized skin.

Psychological uses: Mild depression, apathy.

Subtle uses: Clears energy blocks. Balances energy centers.

Notes: Avoid Eucalyptus, Smithii during pregnancy and nursing.

* Chemical component percentages may vary. Essential 3 offers a *Certificate of Analysis* for review.

Methods of use:

After Shower	Bath
Bath, Foot	Chest Rub
Compress	Diffusion
Inhalation	Inhalation, Hot Water
Massage	Room Mist
Spot Application	Anointing Oil

For more information, see Methods of Using Essential Oils on page xi.

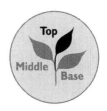

NOTES

Avoid during pregnancy and nursing

Suited for long-term use

Good for children, frail and elderly

Good for preventing colds and flu

Excellent for muscle and joint aches

Which One?

As a whole, the Eucalyptuses are for respiratory congestion and infection, immune support, and muscle aches. Their aromas are strong, refreshing, and camphoraceous. All are more or less stimulating except **Euc. Citriodora.** Choose **Euc. Globulus** for its strength, **Euc. Radiata** for longer-term use and its pleasant aroma, **Euc. Citriodora** for air disinfecting and night-time use, and **Euc. Smithii** for prevention, muscle and joint aches, and its mildness.

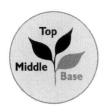

NOTES

*Avoid during pregnancy
and nursing*

Indigestion relief

Anise-like aroma

Fennel, Sweet

Latin name: *Foeniculum vulgare*

Country of origin: Egypt

Part of the plant: Crushed seeds

Extraction method: Steam distilled

Main biochemical components*: Anetheole, limonene, phellandrene

Physical uses: Indigestion, nausea, muscle spasms, intestinal spasms, hiccups, lymphatic support.

Skin care uses: Skin tonic, wrinkles.

Psychological uses: Nervous tension, stress.

Subtle uses: Increases courage and confidence. Motivates.

Notes: Use Fennel, Sweet in a 1-5% dilution. Avoid during pregnancy and nursing.

* Chemical component percentages may vary.
   Essential 3 offers a *Certificate of Analysis* for review.

Methods of use:

Compress	Compress, Facial
Diffusion	Inhalation
Massage	Room Mist
Spot Application	Anointing Oil

For more information, see Methods of Using Essential Oils on page xi.

Fir Needle, Balsam

Latin name: *Abies balsamea*

Country of origin: Canada

Part of the plant: Needles and twigs

Extraction method: Steam distilled

Main biochemical components*: Beta-pinene, delta 3-carene, bornyl acetate

Physical uses: Respiratory congestion, infections, colds, flu, sinusitis, bronchitis, coughs, sore throats, shortness of breath, muscle aches, stiff joints.

Skin care uses: n/a

Psychological uses: Stress, mild depression, anxiety.

Subtle uses: Clears energy blocks. Increases intuition.

Notes: Use Fir Needle, Balsam in a 1-5% dilution.

* Chemical component percentages may vary. Essential 3 offers a *Certificate of Analysis* for review.

Methods of use:

Bath, Foot	Chest Rub
Compress	Diffusion
Inhalation	Massage
Room Mist	Spot Application
Anointing Oil	

For more information, see Methods of Using Essential Oils on page xi.

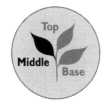

NOTES

Dry coughs

Good anti-inflammatory

Immune support

Which One?

Fir Needle, Balsam has a warm, fresh, woodsy, balsamic aroma. **Fir Needle, Douglas** has a clear, fresh, woodsy, citrusy aroma. They are both warming and good for muscle aches and respiratory congestion. **Balsam** is a good choice for dry coughs. **Douglas** is more complex and offers more immune support. It is also a good air disinfectant.

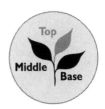

NOTES

Avoid during pregnancy and nursing

Air disinfectant

Immune support

Fir Needle, Douglas

Latin name: *Pseudotsuga menziesii*

Country of origin: Slovenia

Part of the plant: Needles

Extraction method: Steam distilled

Main biochemical components*: Camphene, alpha-pinene, beta-pinene

Physical uses: Respiratory congestion, infections, colds, flu, bronchitis, muscle aches, poor circulation, immune support.

Skin care uses: n/a

Psychological uses: Anxiety, stress, instability, mild depression.

Subtle uses: Clears energy blocks. Grounds and increases intuition.

Notes: Use Fir Needle, Douglas in a 1-5% dilution. Avoid during pregnancy and nursing.

* Chemical component percentages may vary. Essential 3 offers a *Certificate of Analysis* for review.

Methods of use:

Bath, Foot	Chest Rub
Compress	Diffusion
Inhalation	Massage
Room Mist	Spot Application
Anointing Oil	

For more information, see Methods of Using Essential Oils on page xi.

Which One?

Fir Needle, Balsam has a warm, fresh, woodsy, balsamic aroma. **Fir Needle, Douglas** has a clear, fresh, woodsy, citrusy aroma. They are both warming and good for muscle aches and respiratory congestion. **Balsam** is a good choice for dry coughs. **Douglas** is more complex and offers more immune support. It is also a good air disinfectant.

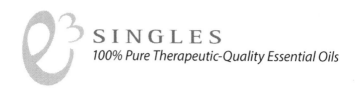
Fragonia

Latin name: *Agonis fragrans*

Country of origin: Australia

Part of the plant: Leaves and flowers

Extraction method: Steam distilled

Main biochemical components*: 1,8 cineol, pinene, linalol, geraniol, terpinen-4-ol

Physical uses: Muscle aches, stiff joints, inflammation, infections (bacterial, fungal), respiratory congestion, immune support.

Skin care uses: Infections (bacterial, fungal), inflammation.

Psychological uses: Sleeplessness, emotional balancer.

Notes: Fragonia is the only essential oil to have a balance of chemical constituents in a near perfect 1:1:1 ratio of monoterpenes, oxides and monoterpenols, which gives it a unique ability to create harmony and balance in the emotional body.

*Chemical component percentages may vary. Essential 3 offers a *Certificate of Analysis* for review.

Methods of use:

After Shower	Bath
Bath, Foot	Chest Rub
Compress, facial	Diffusion
Massage	Inhalation
Room Mist	Scalp Oil
Spot Application	Anointing Oil
Inhalation, Hot Water	

For more information, see Methods of Using Essential Oils on page xi.

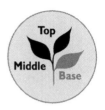

NOTES

Immune support

Emotional balancer

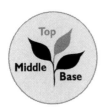
NOTES

Avoid during pregnancy and nursing

Immune stimulant

Stress relief

Skin care

Meditation

Hospice use for transition

Frankincense (Ethiopia)

Latin name: *Boswellia carterii*

Country of origin: Ethiopia

Part of the plant: Resin ("tears")

Extraction method: Steam distilled

Main biochemical components*: Alpha-pinene, limonene, para-cymene

Physical uses: Coughs, bronchitis, inflammation, infections, tense breathing, rapid breathing, shallow breathing, PMS, menopausal symptoms, immune support.

Skin care uses: Wrinkles, dry skin, mature skin, scars, inflammation, small wounds, infections, skin tonic.

Psychological uses: Anxiety, stress, nervous tension, fear, restless mind.

Subtle uses: Quiets and clarifies the mind.

Notes: Avoid Frankincense (Ethiopia) during pregnancy and nursing.

* Chemical component percentages may vary. Essential 3 offers a *Certificate of Analysis* for review.

Methods of use:

Add to Products	After Shower
Bath	Bath, Foot
Body Lotion	Body Oil
Chest Rub	Compress
Compress, Facial	Diffusion
Facial Oil	Inhalation
Inhalation, Hot Water	Massage
Room Mist	Skin Mist
Spot Application	Anointing Oil

For more information, see Methods of Using Essential Oils on page xi.

Which One?

All the Frankincenses have a warm, sweet, balsamic, woody aroma. **Ethiopia** is a little deeper, **Oman** is a little more refreshing, **Somalia** is a little spicier. They are interchangeable in the uses— all being good for stress, skin care, meditation, and as immune stimulants.

Frankincense (Oman)

Latin name: *Boswellia frereana*

Country of origin: Oman

Part of the plant: Resin ("tears")

Extraction method: Steam distilled

Main biochemical components*: Alpha-pinene, beta-pinene, octyl acetate

Physical uses: Coughs, bronchitis, inflammation, infections, tense breathing, shallow breathing, rapid breathing, PMS, menopausal symptoms, immune support.

Skin care uses: Wrinkles, dry skin, mature skin, scars, infections, inflammation, small wounds, skin tonic.

Psychological uses: Anxiety, stress, nervous tension, fear, restless mind.

Subtle uses: Quiets and clarifies the mind.

Notes: Avoid Frankincense (Oman) during pregnancy and nursing.

* Chemical component percentages may vary.
  Essential 3 offers a *Certificate of Analysis* for review.

Methods of use:

Add to Products	After Shower
Bath	Bath, Foot
Body Lotion	Body Oil
Chest Rub	Compress
Compress, Facial	Diffusion
Facial Oil	Inhalation
Inhalation, Hot Water	Massage
Room Mist	Skin Mist
Spot Application	Anointing Oil

For more information, see Methods of Using Essential Oils on page xi.

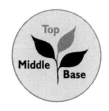

NOTES

Avoid during pregnancy and nursing

Immune stimulant

Stress relief

Skin care

Meditation

Hospice use for transition

Which One?

All the Frankincenses have a warm, sweet, balsamic, woody aroma. **Ethiopia** is a little deeper, **Oman** is a little more refreshing, **Somalia** is a little spicier. They are interchangeable in the uses— all being good for stress, skin care, meditation, and as immune stimulants.

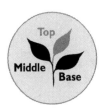

NOTES

Avoid during pregnancy and nursing

Immune stimulant

Stress relief

Skin care

Meditation

Hospice use for transition

Frankincense (Somalia)

Latin name: *Boswellia frereana*

Country of origin: Somalia

Part of the plant: Resin ("tears")

Extraction method: Steam distilled

Main biochemical components*: Alpha-pinene, alpha-phellandrene, para-cymene

Physical uses: Coughs, bronchitis, inflammation, infections, tense breathing, shallow breathing, rapid breathing, PMS, menopausal symptoms, immune support.

Skin care uses: Wrinkles, dry skin, mature skin, scars, inflammation, small wounds, infections, skin tonic.

Psychological uses: Anxiety, stress, nervous tension, fear, restless mind.

Subtle uses: Quiets and clarifies the mind.

Notes: Avoid Frankincense (Somalia) during pregnancy and nursing.

* Chemical component percentages may vary.
  Essential 3 offers a *Certificate of Analysis* for review.

Methods of use:

Add to Products	After Shower
Bath	Bath, Foot
Body Lotion	Body Oil
Chest Rub	Compress
Compress, Facial	Diffusion
Facial Oil	Inhalation
Inhalation, Hot Water	Massage
Room Mist	Skin Mist
Spot Application	Anointing Oil

For more information, see Methods of Using Essential Oils on page xi.

Which One?

All the Frankincenses have a warm, sweet, balsamic, woody aroma. **Ethiopia** is a little deeper, **Oman** is a little more refreshing, **Somalia** is a little spicier. They are interchangeable in the uses—all being good for stress, skin care, meditation, and as immune stimulants.

Geranium (China)

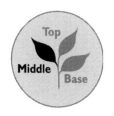

Top
Middle
Base

Latin name: *Pelargonium graveolens*

Country of origin: China

Part of the plant: Leaves

Extraction method: Steam distilled

Main biochemical components*: Citronellol, citronellal formate, geraniol

Physical uses: Infections (bacterial, fungal), sore throats, PMS, menopausal symptoms, poor circulation, circulatory congestion, stiff joints, immune support, lymphatic support, general tonic.

Skin care uses: Imbalanced oil production, poor circulation, small wounds, infections (bacterial, fungal), dermatitis, burns, bruises, eczema, skin tonic.

Psychological uses: Stress, anxiety, mood swings, mild depression.

Subtle uses: Promotes harmony. Nourishes the feminine.

Notes: Avoid Geranium (China) during pregnancy and nursing.

* Chemical component percentages may vary. Essential 3 offers a *Certificate of Analysis* for review.

Methods of use:

Add to Products	After Shower
Bath	Bath, Foot
Body Lotion	Body Oil
Compress	Compress, Facial
Diffusion	Facial Oil
Inhalation	Inhalation, Hot Water
Massage	Room Mist
Skin Mist	Spot Application
Anointing Oil	

For more information, see Methods of Using Essential Oils on page xi.

NOTES

Avoid during pregnancy and nursing

Stress relief

Balancing

Skin care

PMS

Menopause

Adaptogenic

Styptic

Which One?

All the Geraniums have a herbaceous, slightly floral, soft, green aroma. **Geranium (China)** is a little more citrusy, **Geranium (Egypt)** is a little greener, and **Geranium, Rose** is a little more floral (sweeter). They are interchangeable in the uses—all being good for stress, skin care, PMS, and menopause.

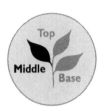

NOTES

Avoid during pregnancy and nursing

Stress relief

Balancing

Skin care

PMS

Menopause

Adaptogenic

Styptic

Which One?

All the Geraniums have a herbaceous, slightly floral, soft, green aroma. **Geranium (China)** is a little more citrusy, **Geranium (Egypt)** is a little greener, and **Geranium, Rose** is a little more floral (sweeter). They are interchangeable in the uses—all being good for stress, skin care, PMS, and menopause.

e³ SINGLES
100% Pure Therapeutic-Quality Essential Oils

Geranium (Egypt)

Latin name: *Pelargonium graveolens*

Country of origin: Egypt

Part of the plant: Leaves

Extraction method: Steam distilled

Main biochemical components*: Citronellol, geraniol, linalol

Physical uses: Infections (bacterial, fungal), respiratory congestion, sore throats, PMS, menopausal symptoms, poor circulation, circulatory congestion, stiff joints, immune support, lymphatic support, general tonic.

Skin care uses: Imbalanced oil production, poor circulation, small wounds, infections (bacterial, fungal), dermatitis, burns, bruises, eczema, skin tonic.

Psychological uses: Stress, anxiety, mood swings, mild depression.

Subtle uses: Promotes harmony. Nourishes the feminine.

Notes: Avoid Geranium (Egypt) during pregnancy and nursing.

* Chemical component percentages may vary. Essential 3 offers a *Certificate of Analysis* for review.

Methods of use:

Add to Products	After Shower
Bath	Bath, Foot
Body Lotion	Body Oil
Compress	Compress, Facial
Diffusion	Facial Oil
Inhalation	Inhalation, Hot Water
Massage	Room Mist
Skin Mist	Spot Application
Anointing Oil	

For more information, see Methods of Using Essential Oils on page xi.

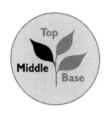

Geranium, Rose

Latin name: *Pelargonium roseum*

Country of origin: Madagascar

Part of the plant: Leaves

Extraction method: Steam distilled

Main biochemical components*: Citronellol, geraniol, linalol

Physical uses: Infections (bacterial, fungal), respiratory congestion, sore throats, PMS, menopausal symptoms, poor circulation, circulatory congestion, stiff joints, immune support, lymphatic support, general tonic.

Skin care uses: Imbalanced oil production, poor circulation, small wounds, infections (bacterial, fungal), dermatitis, burns, bruises, eczema, skin tonic.

Psychological uses: Stress, anxiety, mood swings, mild depression.

Subtle uses: Promotes harmony. Nourishes the feminine.

Notes: Avoid Geranium, Rose during pregnancy and nursing.

* Chemical component percentages may vary. Essential 3 offers a *Certificate of Analysis* for review.

Methods of use:

Add to Products	After Shower
Bath	Bath, Foot
Body Lotion	Body Oil
Compress	Compress, Facial
Diffusion	Facial Oil
Inhalation	Inhalation, Hot Water
Massage	Room Mist
Skin Mist	Spot Application
Anointing Oil	

For more information, see Methods of Using Essential Oils on page xi.

NOTES

Avoid during pregnancy and nursing

Stress relief

Balancing

Skin care

PMS

Menopause

Adaptogenic

Styptic

Which One?

All the Geraniums have a herbaceous, slightly floral, soft, green aroma. **Geranium (China)** is a little more citrusy, **Geranium (Egypt)** is a little greener, and **Geranium, Rose** is a little more floral (sweeter). They are interchangeable in the uses—all being good for stress, skin care, PMS, and menopause.

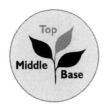

NOTES

Avoid use in sun

Avoid use during

pregnancy

and nursing

Nausea / upset stomach

relief

Aphrodisiac

Ginger

Latin name: *Zingiber officinale*

Country of origin: Madagascar

Part of the plant: Fresh root

Extraction method: Hydro-diffused

Main biochemical components*: Beta-bisabolene, ar-curcumene, camphene

Physical uses: Poor circulation, feeling cold, infections, muscle aches, muscle spasms, menstrual cramps, stiff joints, indigestion, nausea, respiratory congestion, bronchitis.

Skin care uses: n/a

Psychological uses: Nervous exhaustion, mental fatigue, mental fog, emotional coolness, emotional instability, low libido.

Subtle uses: Generally strengthens and stabilizes. Promotes confidence and courage.

Notes: Use Ginger in a 1-5 % dilution. Do not use directly on the skin when you are going to be in the sun. Avoid use during pregnancy and nursing.

* Chemical component percentages may vary. Essential 3 offers a *Certificate of Analysis* for review.

Methods of use:

Bath, Foot	Chest Rub
Compress	Diffusion
Inhalation	Massage (specific area)
Spot Application	Anointing Oil

For more information, see Methods of Using Essential Oils on page xi.

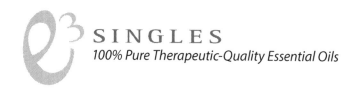
Grapefruit, Red

Latin name: *Citrus paradisi*

Country of origin: USA

Part of the plant: Rinds

Extraction method: Cold pressed

Main biochemical components*: D-limonene, geraniol, cadinene

Physical uses: Poor circulation, muscle fatigue, infections, water retention, lymphatic support, immune support.

Skin care uses: Athlete's foot, oily/congested skin, infections.

Psychological uses: Mental fog, mental fatigue, mild depression, nervous exhaustion.

Subtle uses: Clears energy blocks. Promotes confidence. Increases intuition.

Notes: Do not use Grapefruit, Red directly on the skin when you are going to be in the sun.

* Chemical component percentages may vary. Essential 3 offers a *Certificate of Analysis* for review.

Methods of use:

After Shower	Bath
Bath, Foot	Compress
Compress, Facial	Diffusion
Inhalation	Massage
Room Mist	Spot Application
Anointing Oil	

For more information, see Methods of Using Essential Oils on page xi.

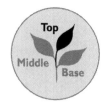

NOTES

Avoid use in sun

Appetite suppressant

Air disinfectant

Uplifting, fresh aroma

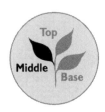

NOTES

Unsurpassed for bruises

Calms nervous system

Helichrysum

Latin name: *Helichrysum italicum*

Country of origin: France

Part of the plant: Flower clusters

Extraction method: Steam distilled

Main biochemical components*: Alpha-pinene, gamma-curcumene, isoprenoid diketones

Physical uses: Bronchitis, sinusitis, coughs, colds, flu, muscle aches, inflammation, infections (bacterial, viral), allergic reactions, stiff joints, poor circulation, nerve pain, lymphatic support, immune support.

Skin care uses: Bruises, scars, infections (bacterial, viral), small wounds, burns, allergic reactions, dermatitis, eczema, inflammation.

Psychological uses: Mild depression, nervous exhaustion, shock.

Subtle uses: Clears energy blocks, especially due to negative emotions. Promotes compassion for others and self.

Notes: Helichrysum is the best essential oil for bruises.

* Chemical component percentages may vary. Essential 3 offers a *Certificate of Analysis* for review.

Methods of use:

After Shower	Bath
Bath, Foot	Chest Rub
Compress	Inhalation
Inhalation, Hot Water	Massage
Spot Application	Anointing Oil

For more information, see Methods of Using Essential Oils on page xi.

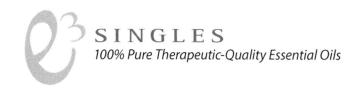
Jasmine

Latin name: *Jasminum officinale* var. *grandiflorum*

Country of origin: India

Part of the plant: Flowers

Extraction method: Absolute

Main biochemical components*: Benzyl benzoate+phytol, benzyl acetate, phytol acetate

Physical uses: Muscle aches, muscle spasms, stiff joints, menstrual cramps, labor cramps.

Skin care uses: Dry skin, irritated skin, skin tonic.

Psychological uses: Nervousness, anxiety, stress, lack of sense of well-being, mild depression, worry, negativity, low libido, sleeplessness.

Subtle uses: Promotes creativity and sensuality. Eases grief and heartache. Inspires.

Notes: Use Jasmine in a 1-5 % dilution. Avoid during pregnancy and nursing.

* Chemical component percentages may vary. Essential 3 offers a *Certificate of Analysis* for review.

Methods of use:

Add to Products	After Shower
Bath	Bath, Foot
Body Lotion	Body Oil
Compress	Compress, Facial
Diffusion	Facial Oil
Inhalation	Massage
Perfume	Skin Mist
Spot Application	Anointing Oil

For more information, see Methods of Using Essential Oils on page xi.

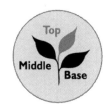

NOTES

Avoid during pregnancy and nursing

Premier aphrodisiac

Favorite perfume

Sleep aid

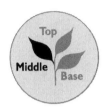

Top
Middle
Base

NOTES

Avoid during pregnancy and nursing

Avoid w/kidney conditions

Stimulant

Air disinfectant

Juniper Berry

Latin name: *Juniperus communis*

Country of origin: Bosnia

Part of the plant: Berries only (dried/partially dried)

Extraction method: Steam distilled

Main biochemical components*: Alpha-pinene, sabinene, limonene

Physical uses: Poor circulation, infections, colds, flu, stiff joints, fatigue, immune support, lymphatic support.

Skin care uses: Blemishes, oily skin, infections, clogged pores, astringent.

Psychological uses: Anxiety, mild depression, mental fog.

Subtle uses: Clears energy blocks and negativity. Strengthens will power and promotes confidence.

Notes: Use Juniper Berry in a 1-5 % dilution. It can have a diuretic effect, so it is not recommended for someone who has kidney disease or infection. Avoid during pregnancy and nursing.

* Chemical component percentages may vary. Essential 3 offers a *Certificate of Analysis* for review.

Methods of use:

Bath	Bath, Foot
Chest Rub	Compress
Diffusion	Inhalation
Massage	Room Mist
Spot Application	Anointing Oil

For more information, see Methods of Using Essential Oils on page xi.

Which One?
The Junipers have a clear, sharp, fresh, woody aroma. **Juniper Berry** is slightly drier and sharper. **Juniperberry** is slightly sweeter and softer. They are interchangeable in their uses—both being stimulating, good for lymphatic and immune support, and effective air disinfectants.

Juniperberry

Latin name: *Juniperus communis*

Country of origin: Russia

Part of the plant: Berries (dried/partially dried) and twigs

Extraction method: Steam distilled

Main biochemical components*: Pinene, myrcene, limonene

Physical uses: Poor circulation, infections, colds, flu, stiff joints, fatigue, immune support, lymphatic support.

Skin care uses: Blemishes, oily skin, infections, clogged pores, astringent.

Psychological uses: Anxiety, mild depression, mental fog.

Subtle uses: Clears energy blocks and negativity. Strengthens will power and promotes confidence.

Notes: Use Juniperberry in a 1-5% dilution. It can have a diuretic effect, so it is not recommended for someone who has kidney disease or infection. Avoid during pregnancy and nursing.

* Chemical component percentages may vary. Essential 3 offers a *Certificate of Analysis* for review.

Methods of use:

Bath	Bath, Foot
Chest Rub	Compress
Diffusion	Inhalation
Massage	Room Mist
Spot Application	Anointing Oil

For more information, see Methods of Using Essential Oils on page xi.

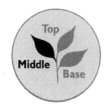

NOTES

Avoid during pregnancy and nursing

Avoid w/kidney conditions

Stimulant

Air disinfectant

Which One?

The Junipers have a clear, sharp, fresh, woody aroma. **Juniper Berry** is slightly drier and sharper. **Juniperberry** is slightly sweeter and softer. They are interchangeable in their uses—both being stimulating, good for lymphatic and immune support, and effective air disinfectants.

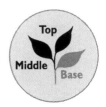

Top
Middle
Base

NOTES

Exceptionally versatile

Stress relief

Skin care

Excellent for burns

Sleep aid

Adaptogenic

Which One?

The true lavenders (*Lavandula angustifolia*) have a fresh, sweet, soft, herbaceous/floral aroma. The Lavenders from **Bulgaria** and **France** are a little sweeter and softer, and the **Organic** is a little fresher. They are interchangeable in their uses—being versatile, and good for skin care and the nervous system. **Lavender, Spike** has a fresh, sharp, herbaceous aroma. Choose **Spike** for respiratory and muscle conditions, and for immune support.

Lavender (Bulgaria)

Latin name: *Lavandula angustifolia*

Country of origin: Bulgaria

Part of the plant: Flowering tops

Extraction method: Steam distilled

Main biochemical components*: Linalyl acetate, linalol, (Z)-beta-ocimene

Physical uses: Respiratory congestion, bronchitis, laryngitis, colds, flu, tense breathing, muscle spasms, muscle aches, muscle cramps, infections (bacterial, viral), headaches, inflammation, lymphatic support.

Skin care uses: Imbalanced oil production, small wounds, bruises, burns, sunburn, insect bites and stings, infections (bacterial, viral), inflammation, irritations, itching, blemishes, eczema, skin tonic.

Psychological uses: Stress, nervous tension, anxiety, nervous exhaustion, mood swings, anger, sleeplessness.

Subtle uses: Balances the energy centers. Calms. Clears energy blocks. Brings in positive energy.

Notes: Lavender is one of the most versatile essential oils.

* Chemical component percentages may vary. Essential 3 offers a *Certificate of Analysis* for review.

Methods of use:

Add to Products	After Shower	Bath
Bath, Foot	Body Lotion	Body Oil
Chest Rub	Compress	Compress, Facial
Diffusion	Facial Oil	Inhalation
Inhalation, Hot Water	Massage	Room Mist
Skin Mist	Spot Application	Anointing Oil

For more information, see Methods of Using Essential Oils on page xi.

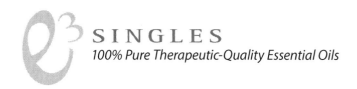

Lavender (France, High Altitude)

Latin name: *Lavandula angustifolia*

Country of origin: France

Part of the plant: Flowering tops

Extraction method: Steam distilled

Main biochemical components*: Linalyl acetate, linalol, (E)-anethole

Physical uses: Respiratory congestion, bronchitis, laryngitis, colds, flu, tense breathing, muscle spasms, muscle aches, muscle cramps, infections (bacterial, viral) headaches, inflammation, lymphatic support.

Skin care uses: Imbalanced oil production, small wounds, bruises, burns, sunburn, insect bites and stings, infections (bacterial, viral), irritations, inflammation, itching, blemishes, eczema, skin tonic.

Psychological uses: Stress, nervous tension, anxiety, nervous exhaustion, mood swings, anger, sleeplessness.

Subtle uses: Balances the energy centers. Calms. Clears energy blocks. Brings in positive energy.

Notes: Lavender is one of the most versatile essential oils. The French, high-altitude Lavender is one of the most prized lavenders, known for its exquisite aroma and superb relaxing qualities.

* Chemical component percentages may vary. Essential 3 offers a *Certificate of Analysis* for review.

Methods of use:

Add to Products	After Shower	Bath
Bath, Foot	Body Lotion	Body Oil
Chest Rub	Compress	Compress, Facial
Diffusion	Facial Oil	Inhalation
Inhalation, Hot Water	Massage	Room Mist
Skin Mist	Spot Application	Anointing Oil

For more information, see Methods of Using Essential Oils on page xi.

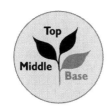

NOTES

Exceptionally versatile

Stress relief

Skin care

Excellent for burns

Hospital comfort care

Sleep aid

Adaptogenic

Which One?

The true lavenders (*Lavandula angustifolia*) have a fresh, sweet, soft, herbaceous/floral aroma. The Lavenders from **Bulgaria** and **France** are a little sweeter and softer, and the **Organic** is a little fresher. They are interchangeable in their uses—being versatile, and good for skin care and the nervous system. **Lavender, Spike** has a fresh, sharp, herbaceous aroma. Choose **Spike** for respiratory and muscle conditions, and for immune support.

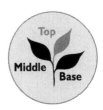

NOTES

Exceptionally versatile

Stress relief

Skin care

Excellent for burns

Sleep aid

Adaptogenic

Lavender, Organic

Latin name: *Lavandula angustifolia*

Country of origin: USA

Part of the plant: Flowering tops

Extraction method: Steam distilled

Main biochemical components*: Linalyl acetate, linalol, (Z)-beta-ocimene

Physical uses: Respiratory congestion, bronchitis, laryngitis, colds, flu, tense breathing, muscle spasms, muscle aches, muscle cramps, infections (bacterial, viral) headaches, inflammation, lymphatic support.

Skin care uses: Imbalanced oil production, small wounds, bruises, burns, sunburn, insect bites and stings, infections (bacterial, viral), irritations, inflammation, itching, blemishes, eczema, skin tonic.

Psychological uses: Stress, nervous tension, anxiety, nervous exhaustion, mood swings, anger, sleeplessness.

Subtle uses: Balances the energy centers. Calms. Clears energy blocks. Brings in positive energy.

Notes: Lavender is one of the most versatile essential oils.

* Chemical component percentages may vary. Essential 3 offers a *Certificate of Analysis* for review.

Methods of use:

Add to Products	After Shower	Bath
Bath, Foot	Body Lotion	Body Oil
Chest Rub	Compress	Compress, Facial
Diffusion	Facial Oil	Inhalation
Inhalation, Hot Water	Massage	Room Mist
Skin Mist	Spot Application	Anointing Oil

For more information, see Methods of Using Essential Oils on page xi.

Which One?

The true lavenders (*Lavandula angustifolia*) have a fresh, sweet, soft, herbaceous/floral aroma. The Lavenders from **Bulgaria** and **France** are a little sweeter and softer, and the **Organic** is a little fresher. They are interchangeable in their uses—being versatile, and good for skin care and the nervous system. **Lavender, Spike** has a fresh, sharp, herbaceous aroma. Choose **Spike** for respiratory and muscle conditions, and for immune support.

Lavender, Spike

Latin name: *Lavandula latifolia*

Country of origin: France

Part of the plant: Flowering tops

Extraction method: Steam distilled

Main biochemical components*: Linalol, 1,8 cineole, camphor

Physical uses: Respiratory congestion, bronchitis, sinusitis, sore throat, cough, tonsillitis, colds, flu, infections, muscle aches, stiff joints, headaches, immune support.

Skin care uses: Blemishes, insect bites and stings, small wounds, burns, infections.

Psychological uses: Mental fatigue, mental fog.

Subtle uses: Clears energy blocks. Brings in positive energy.

Notes: Avoid Lavender, Spike with high blood pressure. Avoid during pregnancy and nursing.

* Chemical component percentages may vary. Essential 3 offers a *Certificate of Analysis* for review.

Methods of use:

After Shower	Bath
Bath, Foot	Chest Rub
Compress	Diffusion
Inhalation	Inhalation, Hot Water
Massage	Room Mist
Spot Application	Anointing Oil

For more information, see Methods of Using Essential Oils on page xi.

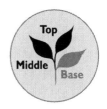

NOTES

Avoid w/ high
blood pressure
Avoid during pregnancy
and nursing
Immune stimulant
For massage: 1 drop on
tissue, underside of face
cradle to relieve
face-pressure stuffiness

Which One?

The true lavenders (*Lavandula angustifolia*) have a fresh, sweet, soft, herbaceous/floral aroma. The Lavenders from **Bulgaria** and **France** are a little sweeter and softer, and the **Organic** is a little fresher. They are interchangeable in their uses—being versatile, and good for skin care and the nervous system. **Lavender, Spike** has a fresh, sharp, herbaceous aroma. Choose **Spike** for respiratory and muscle conditions, and for immune support.

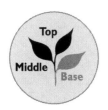

NOTES

Avoid use in sun

Immune stimulant

Air disinfectant (especially for sick rooms)

Liver detox

Uplifting, bright aroma

Lemon

Latin name: *Citrus limonum*

Country of origin: Italy

Part of the plant: Rinds

Extraction method: Cold pressed

Main biochemical components*: Limonene, beta-pinene, gamma-terpinene

Physical uses: Infections (bacterial, fungal, viral), sinusitis, colds, flu, sore throat, poor circulation, immune support.

Skin care uses: Congested skin, oily skin, blemishes, infections (bacterial, fungal, viral), imbalanced oil production, warts, skin tonic.

Psychological uses: Mental fog, mental clarity, mild depression.

Subtle uses: Clears energy blocks. Clears emotional confusion. Promotes mental clarity and objectivity.

Notes: Use Lemon in a 1-5% dilution. Do not use directly on the skin when you are going to be in the sun.

* Chemical component percentages may vary.
   Essential 3 offers a *Certificate of Analysis* for review.

Methods of use:

After Shower	Bath
Bath, Foot	Chest Rub
Compress	Compress, Facial
Diffusion	Inhalation
Inhalation, Hot Water	Massage
Room Mist	Spot Application
Anointing Oil	

For more information, see Methods of Using Essential Oils on page xi.

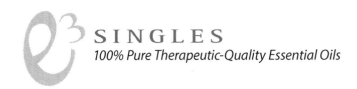

SINGLES
100% Pure Therapeutic-Quality Essential Oils

Lemongrass

Latin name: *Cymbopogon flexuosus*

Country of origin: India

Part of the plant: Leaves (fresh/partially dried)

Extraction method: Steam distilled

Main biochemical components*: Geranial, neral, geraniol

Physical uses: Muscle aches, muscle fatigue, stiff joints, jet lag, poor circulation, indigestion, infections, lymphatic support, immune support.

Skin care uses: Congested skin, oily skin, blemishes, infections, nail fungus, athlete's foot, body odor, bruises, skin tonic.

Psychological uses: Stress, anxiety, nervous exhaustion, mental fatigue, mental fog, mild depression.

Subtle uses: Clears energy blocks. Dispels negativity.

Notes: Use Lemongrass in a 1-5% dilution. May be sensitizing. Avoid during pregnancy and nursing.

* Chemical component percentages may vary. Essential 3 offers a *Certificate of Analysis* for review.

Methods of use:

After Shower	Bath, Foot
Compress	Diffusion
Inhalation	Massage
Room Mist	Spot Application
Anointing Oil	

For more information, see Methods of Using Essential Oils on page xi.

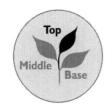

NOTES

May be sensitizing

Avoid during pregnancy and nursing

Muscle ache compress (1 drop in water)

Bright, lemony aroma

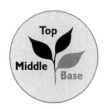

SINGLES
100% Pure Therapeutic-Quality Essential Oils

Top
Middle
Base

NOTES

May be sensitizing

Avoid use in sun

Uplifting, bright aroma

Lime

Latin name: *Citrus aurantifolia*

Country of origin: Brazil

Part of the plant: Rinds

Extraction method: Cold pressed

Main biochemical components*: Limonene, pinene, terpinene

Physical uses: Respiratory congestion, coughs, colds, sore throat, infections, muscle spasms, immune support.

Skin care uses: Body odor, oily skin, infections.

Psychological uses: Mild depression, apathy, anxiety, mental fatigue.

Subtle uses: Clears energy blocks. Clears the mind.

Notes: Use Lime in a 1-5% dilution. May be sensitizing. Do not use directly on the skin when you are going to be in the sun.

* Chemical component percentages may vary.
   Essential 3 offers a *Certificate of Analysis* for review.

Methods of use:

Bath, Foot	Chest Rub
Compress	Diffusion
Inhalation	Massage
Room Mist	Spot Application
Anointing Oil	

For more information, see Methods of Using Essential Oils on page xi.

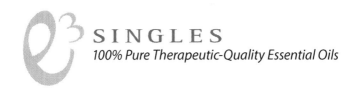

Mandarin, Red

Latin name: *Citrus deliciosa*

Country of origin: Italy

Part of the plant: Rinds

Extraction method: Cold pressed

Main biochemical components*: Limonene, gamma-terpinene, para-cymene

Physical uses: Indigestion, tense breathing, muscle spasms, PMS, lymphatic support, immune support.

Skin care uses: Congested skin, oily skin, blemished skin, dry skin, rough skin, scars, skin tonic.

Psychological uses: Stress, anxiety, mild depression, tension, restlessness, sleeplessness.

Subtle uses: Promotes joy and happiness. Inspires.

Notes: Do not use Mandarin, Red directly on the skin when you are going to be in the sun.

* Chemical component percentages may vary. Essential 3 offers a *Certificate of Analysis* for review.

Methods of use:

After Shower	Bath
Bath, Foot	Chest Rub
Compress	Compress, Facial
Diffusion	Inhalation
Massage	Room Mist
Spot Application	Anointing Oil

For more information, see Methods of Using Essential Oils on page xi.

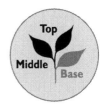

NOTES

Avoid use in sun

Stress relief

A gentle citrus

Uplifting, happy aroma

Sleep aid

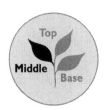

NOTES

A gentle Thyme
Warming for massage

Marjoram, Spanish

Latin name: *Thymus mastichina*

Country of origin: Spain

Part of the plant: Flowering tops and dried leaves

Extraction method: Steam distilled

Main biochemical components*: 1,8 cineole, linalol, alpha-terpineol

Physical uses: Respiratory congestion, sinusitis, colds, bronchitis, infections (viral, bacterial), muscle aches, feeling cold, immune support.

Skin care uses: n/a

Psychological uses: Mental fatigue, mental clarity.

Subtle uses: Clears energy blocks. Promotes self-confidence.

Notes: Use Marjoram, Spanish in a 1-5% dilution.

* Chemical component percentages may vary. Essential 3 offers a *Certificate of Analysis* for review.

Methods of use:

After Shower	Chest Rub
Compress	Diffusion
Inhalation	Massage
Room Mist	Spot Application
Anointing Oil	

For more information, see Methods of Using Essential Oils on page xi.

Which One?

Marjoram, Spanish has a warm, spicy, camphoraceous aroma. It is good for infections, muscle aches, and immune support. It is not a true marjoram and does not have the calming qualities associated with a true marjoram. **Marjoram, Sweet** has a warm, woody-spicy, fresh, herbaceous aroma. It is a true marjoram. It is good for muscle spasms, stress, and insomnia.

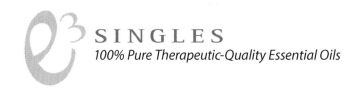

SINGLES
100% Pure Therapeutic-Quality Essential Oils

Marjoram, Sweet

Latin name: *Origanum majorana*

Country of origin: Egypt

Part of the plant: Flowering tops and dried leaves

Extraction method: Steam distilled

Main biochemical components*: Terpinen-4-ol, terpineol, linalyl acetate

Physical uses: Muscle aches, muscle spasms, stiff joints, menstrual cramps, PMS, infections, colds, flu, sinusitis, bronchitis, coughing spasms, tense breathing, constipation, nerve pain, headaches.

Skin care uses: Bruises, small wounds, infections.

Psychological uses: Stress, tension, irritability, trauma, mild depression, restlessness, sleeplessness, too high libido.

Subtle uses: Comforts, especially for grief and loneliness. Promotes confidence and courage. Helps to accept emotional loss.

Notes: Avoid Marjoram, Sweet during pregnancy and nursing.

* Chemical component percentages may vary. Essential 3 offers a *Certificate of Analysis* for review.

Methods of use:

After Shower	Bath
Bath, Foot	Chest Rub
Compress	Diffusion
Inhalation	Inhalation, Hot Water
Massage	Room Mist
Spot Application	Anointing Oil

For more information, see Methods of Using Essential Oils on page xi.

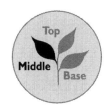

NOTES

Avoid during pregnancy and nursing
Stress relief
Sleep aid

_____

_____

_____

_____

_____

_____

_____

Which One?
Marjoram, Spanish has a warm, spicy, camphoraceous aroma. It is good for infections, muscle aches, and immune support. It is not a true marjoram and does not have the calming qualities associated with a true marjoram. **Marjoram, Sweet** has a warm, woody-spicy, fresh, herbaceous aroma. It is a true marjoram. It is good for muscle spasms, stress, and insomnia.

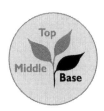

NOTES

Avoid during pregnancy
and nursing
Loss of appetite
Meditation
A drop in mouthwash
blend

Myrrh

Latin name: *Commiphora myrrha*

Country of origin: Ethiopia

Part of the plant: Resin

Extraction method: Steam distilled

Main biochemical components*: Limonene, pinene, eugenol

Physical uses: Bronchitis, coughs, sore throats, infections, mouth and gum disorders, immune support.

Skin care uses: Irritations, chapped skin, dry skin, small wounds (especially chronic), eczema, infections.

Psychological uses: Anxiety, tension, emotional coolness, apathy.

Subtle uses: Strengthens and grounds. Supports spirituality.

Notes: Use Myrrh in a 1-5% dilution. Avoid during pregnancy and nursing.

* Chemical component percentages may vary. Essential 3 offers a *Certificate of Analysis* for review.

Methods of use:

After Shower	Bath
Bath, Foot	Body Lotion
Body Oil	Chest Rub
Diffusion	Inhalation
Inhalation, Hot Water	Massage
Skin Mist	Spot Application
Anointing Oil	

For more information, see Methods of Using Essential Oils on page xi.

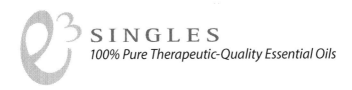
Neroli

Latin name: *Citrus aurantium*

Country of origin: Tunisia

Part of the plant: Flowers (freshly picked)

Extraction method: Steam distilled

Main biochemical components*: Linalol, limonene, beta-pinene

Physical uses: Muscle spasms, poor circulation, nerve pain, intestinal spasms, muscle tonic, infections, immune support.

Skin care uses: Devitalized skin, sun-damaged skin, mature skin, dry skin, sensitive skin, scars, infections, body odor, skin tonic.

Psychological uses: Anxiety, stress, shock, mild depression, sleeplessness, low libido, lack of sense of well-being.

Subtle uses: Brings in positive energy. Eases grief. Promotes feelings of love, peace, lightness and joy.

Notes: Neroli is one of the best essential oils for anxiety.

* Chemical component percentages may vary. Essential 3 offers a *Certificate of Analysis* for review.

Methods of use:

Add to Products	After Shower
Bath	Bath, Foot
Body Lotion	Body Oil
Compress	Compress, Facial
Diffusion	Facial Oil
Inhalation	Massage
Perfume	Room Mist
Skin Mist	Spot Application
Anointing Oil	

For more information, see Methods of Using Essential Oils on page xi.

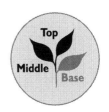

NOTES

Superb for anxiety

Stress relief

Skin care

Aphrodisiac

Sleep aid

Unique, floral aroma

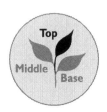

NOTES

Avoid during pregnancy and nursing

Highly anti-infectious

May help protect skin from radiation burns

Hemorrhoid relief (shrinks and soothes)

Niaouli, MQV

Latin name: *Melaleuca quinquenervia*

Country of origin: Spain

Part of the plant: Leaves

Extraction method: Steam distilled

Main biochemical components*: 1,8 cineole, terpineol, pinene

Physical uses: Respiratory congestion, infections (bacterial, viral, fungal), colds, flu, coughs, bronchitis, sore throats, muscle aches, stiff joints, fatigue, poor circulation, immune support, hemorrhoid relief.

Skin care uses: Infections (bacterial, viral, fungal), blemishes, small cuts, insect bites.

Psychological uses: Mental fatigue, mental fog.

Subtle uses: Protects against negativity.

Notes: Avoid Niaouli, MQV during pregnancy and nursing.

* Chemical component percentages may vary. Essential 3 offers a *Certificate of Analysis* for review.

Methods of use:

After Shower	Bath
Bath, Foot	Chest Rub
Compress	Diffusion
Inhalation	Inhalation, Hot Water
Massage	Room Mist
Spot Application	
Anointing Oil	

For more information, see Methods of Using Essential Oils on page xi.

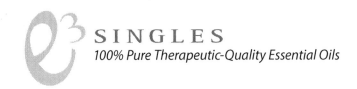

SINGLES
100% Pure Therapeutic-Quality Essential Oils

Nutmeg

Latin name: *Myristica fragrans*

Country of origin: Indonesia

Part of the plant: Seed (dried)

Extraction method: Steam distilled

Main biochemical components*: Sabinene, alpha-pinene, beta-pinene

Physical uses: Muscle aches, muscle spasms, joint stiffness, inflammation, infections (bacterial) feeling cold, poor circulation, general fatigue, nerve pain, poor digestion, indigestion, nausea.

Skin care uses: n/a

Psychological uses: Nervous fatigue, mental fatigue, low libido.

Subtle uses: Increases creativity.

Notes: Use Nutmeg in a 1-5% dilution. Avoid during pregnancy and nursing.

* Chemical component percentages may vary. Essential 3 offers a *Certificate of Analysis* for review.

Methods of use:
Compress
Inhalation
Massage (specific area)
Spot application
Anointing Oil

For more information, see Methods of Using Essential Oils on page xi.

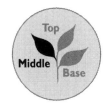

NOTES

Avoid during pregnancy and nursing

Aphrodisiac

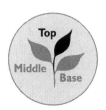

Top

Middle

Base

NOTES

Avoid use in sun

Uplifting, happy aroma

Air freshener

Household cleanser

Which One?

The Oranges have a refreshing, sweet citrus aroma. Orange from the **Dominican Republic** is richer and more complex. **Orange, Sweet** is tangier. Their uses are interchangeable—being good for lymphatic support, uplifting moods, and refreshing the air.

Orange (Dominican Republic)

Latin name: *Citrus sinensis*

Country of origin: Dominican Republic

Part of the plant: Rinds

Extraction method: Cold pressed

Main biochemical components*: Limonene, myrcene, decanal

Physical uses: Poor circulation, poor digestion, water retention, constipation, infections (bacterial, fungal), lymphatic support.

Skin care uses: Dull skin, oily skin, puffy skin, dry skin, wrinkles, rough skin, poor circulation, infections (bacterial, fungal), skin tonic.

Psychological uses: Nervous tension, mild depression, worry, mental fatigue.

Subtle uses: Brings in positive energy. Promotes joy.

Notes: Use Orange (Dominical Republic) in a 1-5% dilution. Do not use directly on the skin when you are going to be in the sun.

* Chemical component percentages may vary. Essential 3 offers a *Certificate of Analysis* for review.

Methods of use:

After Shower	Bath
Bath, Foot	Compress
Compress, Facial	Diffusion
Inhalation	Massage
Room Mist	Spot Application
Anointing Oil	

For more information, see Methods of Using Essential Oils on page xi.

Orange, Sweet

Latin name: *Citrus sinensis*

Country of origin: Portugal

Part of the plant: Rinds

Extraction method: Cold pressed

Main biochemical components*: Limonene, delta-3-carene, linalol

Physical uses: Poor circulation, poor digestion, water retention, constipation, infections (bacterial, fungal), lymphatic support.

Skin care uses: Dull skin, oily skin, puffy skin, dry skin, wrinkles, rough skin, poor circulation, infections (bacterial, fungal), skin tonic.

Psychological uses: Nervous tension, mild depression, worry, mental fatigue.

Subtle uses: Brings in positive energy. Promotes joy.

Notes: Use Orange, Sweet in a 1-5% dilution. Do not use directly on the skin when you are going to be in the sun.

* Chemical component percentages may vary. Essential 3 offers a *Certificate of Analysis* for review.

Methods of use:

After Shower	Bath
Bath, Foot	Compress
Compress, Facial	Diffusion
Inhalation	Massage
Room Mist	Spot Application
Anointing Oil	

For more information, see Methods of Using Essential Oils on page xi.

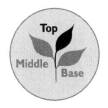

NOTES

Avoid use in sun

Uplifting, happy aroma

Air freshener

Household cleanser

Which One?

The Oranges have a refreshing, sweet citrus aroma. Orange from the **Dominican Republic** is richer and more complex. **Orange, Sweet** is tangier. Their uses are interchangeable—being good for lymphatic support, uplifting moods, and refreshing the air.

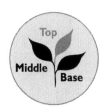

SINGLES
100% Pure Therapeutic-Quality Essential Oils

NOTES

*Avoid use during
pregnancy and nursing
Highly anti-infectious*

Oregano

Latin name: *Origanum vulgare*

Country of origin: Turkey

Part of the plant: Leaves and flowers

Extraction method: Steam distilled

Main biochemical components*: Carvacrol, para-cymene, gamma-gerpinene

Physical uses: Infections (bacterial, fungal), muscle aches, stiff joints, colds, flu, bronchitis, immune support.

Skin care uses: Infections (bacterial, fungal).

Psychological uses: Mental fatigue.

Subtle uses: Promotes mental objectivity and focus.

Notes: Use Oregano in a 1-5% dilution. Avoid during pregnancy and nursing.

* Chemical component percentages may vary. Essential 3 offers a *Certificate of Analysis* for review.

Methods of use:

Chest Rub	Inhalation
Massage (specific area)	Spot Application
Anointing Oil	

For more information, see Methods of Using Essential Oils on page xi.

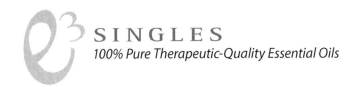

Palmarosa

Latin name: *Cymbopogon martinii*

Country of origin: Nepal

Part of the plant: Grass (fresh or dried)

Extraction method: Steam distilled

Main biochemical components*: Geraniol, geranyl acetate, linalol

Physical uses: Infections (bacterial, viral, fungal), sinusitis, bronchitis, sore throats, poor circulation, chronic fatigue, digestive tonic, muscle tonic, immune support, neuralgia, sciatica, rheumatic pain.

Skin care uses: Imbalanced oil production, dermatitis, infections (bacterial, viral, fungal), devitalized skin, dry skin, wrinkles.

Psychological uses: Nervous exhaustion, stress, anxiety, irritability, mild depression, mental fog.

Subtle uses: Supports physical, emotional, mental, spiritual well-being. Promotes a sense of security. Comforts the heart. Clears the mind. Promotes wisdom.

Notes: Palmarosa is one of the most effective antiviral and antifungal essential oils.

* Chemical component percentages may vary. Essential 3 offers a *Certificate of Analysis* for review.

Methods of use:

Add to Products	After Shower	Bath, Foot
Body Lotion	Body Oil	Chest Rub
Compress	Compress, Facial	Diffusion
Facial Oil	Inhalation	Inhalation, Hot
Water	Massage	Skin Mist
Spot Application	Anointing Oil	

For more information, see Methods of Using Essential Oils on page xi.

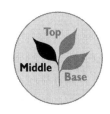

NOTES

Highly anti-infectious

Stress relief

Skin care

Toenail fungus

Geranium-like aroma

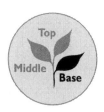

N O T E S

Appetite suppressant

Skin care

Aphrodisiac

Grounding

Distinctive, earthy aroma

Patchouli

Latin name: *Pogostemon cablin*

Country of origin: India

Part of the plant: Leaves

Extraction method: Steam distilled (in iron)

Main biochemical components*: Patchoulol, alpha-balnesene, seychellene

Physical uses: Tense breathing, rapid breathing, infections, water retention.

Skin care uses: Cracked skin, dry skin, devitalized skin, wrinkles, inflammation, dandruff, dermatitis, body odor, infections, small wounds, athlete's foot, skin tonic.

Psychological uses: Nervous exhaustion, stress, lethargy, mood swings, mild depression, low libido.

Subtle uses: Grounds and strengthens. Promotes creativity. Relaxes an over-active intellect.

Notes: Patchouli's aroma has been used to help curb the appetite.

* Chemical component percentages may vary. Essential 3 offers a *Certificate of Analysis* for review.

Methods of use:

Add to Products	After Shower
Bath	Bath, Foot
Body Lotion	Body Oil
Chest Rub	Compress
Compress, Facial	Diffusion
Facial Oil	Inhalation
Perfume	Room Mist
Skin Mist	Scalp Oil
Spot Application	Anointing Oil

For more information, see Methods of Using Essential Oils on page xi.

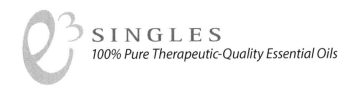
Peppermint

Latin name: *Mentha piperita*

Country of origin: USA

Part of the plant: Leaves, stems, flowers

Extraction method: Steam distilled

Main biochemical components*: Menthol, menthone, isomenthone

Physical uses: Poor digestion, indigestion, nausea, stomach aches, motion sickness, respiratory congestion, sinusitis, coughs, infections (bacterial, viral), muscle aches, muscle spasms, sciatica, stiff joints, menstrual cramps, headaches, feeling over-heated, nerve pain, sluggishness, lymphatic support, immune support.

Skin care uses: Dermatitis, blemishes, infections (bacterial, viral), itching, greasy skin, over-heated skin, rough skin, insect bites and stings.

Psychological uses: Mental fatigue, mental fog, inability to concentrate, anger, nervous stress, mild depression, shock.

Subtle uses: Promotes clarity in communication. Supports a healthy self-esteem. Promotes inspiration and insights.

Notes: Use Peppermint in a 1-5% dilution. May be sensitizing. Avoid during pregnancy and nursing. Do not use with children under 3 years of age.

* Chemical component percentages may vary. Essential 3 offers a *Certificate of Analysis* for review.

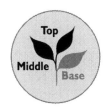

NOTES

May be sensitizing

Avoid during pregnancy and nursing

Do not use with children under 3 years of age

Versatile

Stimulant

Air freshener

Upset stomach

Uplifting, fresh, clean aroma

May not be compatible with homeopathics

Methods of use:

After Shower	Bath, Foot	Chest Rub
Compress	Diffusion	Inhalation
Inhalation, Hot Water	Massage	Room Mist
Skin Mist	Spot Application	Anointing Oil

For more information, see Methods of Using Essential Oils on page xi.

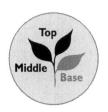

Top
Middle
Base

NOTES

Stress relief

Good in perfume blends

Sleep aid

Petitgrain (Paraguay)

Latin name: *Citrus aurantium*

Country of origin: Paraguay

Part of the plant: Leaves

Extraction method: Steam distilled

Main biochemical components*: Geraniol, limonene, nerol

Physical uses: Tense breathing, muscle spasms, stiff joints, infections (bacterial), inflammation, indigestion, muscle tonic, digestive tonic, immune support.

Skin care uses: Inflammation, infections (bacterial), body odor, skin tonic.

Psychological uses: Stress, anxiety, tension, mental fatigue, mental fog, nervous exhaustion, panic, sleeplessness, mild depression.

Subtle uses: Brings in positive energy. Promotes optimism. Promotes clear perception.

Notes: Petitgrain (Paraguay) is one of the best essential oils for anxiety.

* Chemical component percentages may vary.
  Essential 3 offers a *Certificate of Analysis* for review.

Methods of use:

After Shower	Bath
Bath, Foot	Body Lotion
Body Oil	Chest Rub
Compress	Compress, Facial
Diffusion	Facial Oil
Inhalation	Inhalation, Hot Water
Massage	Room Mist
Skin Mist	Spot Application
Anointing Oil	

For more information, see Methods of Using Essential Oils on page xi.

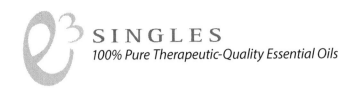
Pine Needle

Latin name: *Pinus sylvestris*

Country of origin: Bulgaria

Part of the plant: Needles

Extraction method: Steam distilled

Main biochemical components*: Alpha-pinene, beta-pinene, para-cymene

Physical uses: Respiratory congestion, sinusitis, colds, flu, bronchitis, sore throat, infections (bacterial, fungal), muscle aches, stiff joints, poor circulation, water retention, fatigue, adrenal support, immune support.

Skin care uses: Congested skin, eczema, minor cuts, infections (bacterial, fungal), body odor, "smoker's skin."

Psychological uses: Mental fatigue, nervous exhaustion.

Subtle uses: Clears energy blocks. Dispels negative energy. Promotes self-confidence and will power. Increases energy in the subtle bodies.

Notes: Use Pine Needle in a 1-5% dilution. May be sensitizing.

* Chemical component percentages may vary. Essential 3 offers a *Certificate of Analysis* for review.

Methods of use:

After Shower	Bath
Bath, Foot	Chest Rub
Compress	Diffusion
Inhalation	Inhalation, Hot Water
Massage	Room Mist
Skin Mist	Spot Application
Anointing Oil	

For more information, see Methods of Using Essential Oils on page xi.

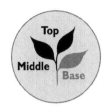

NOTES

May be sensitizing

Stimulant

Adrenal support

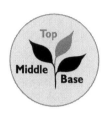

NOTES

Avoid during pregnancy
and nursing
Long-lasting pain relief
Popular in blends for
Thai massage

Plai

Latin name: *Zingiber cassumunar*

Country of origin: Thailand

Part of the plant: Root

Extraction method: Steam distilled

Main biochemical components*: Sabinene, terpineol, zingiberol

Physical uses: Muscle and joint aches, nerve pain, inflammation, infections (bacterial), muscle spasms, menstrual cramps, respiratory congestion, fevers, indigestion, irritated bowels, poor circulation, constipation, diarrhea, nausea.

Skin care uses: Bruises, blemishes, infections (bacterial), inflammation, insect bites.

Psychological uses: Nervousness, anxiety, anger.

Subtle uses: Supports creative thinking. Promotes appreciation. Promotes recovery from trauma.

Notes: Use Plai in a 1-5% dilution. Avoid during pregnancy and nursing.

* Chemical component percentages may vary. Essential 3 offers a *Certificate of Analysis* for review.

Methods of use:

After Shower	Bath
Bath, Foot	Chest Rub
Compress	Diffusion
Inhalation	Inhalation, Hot Water
Massage	Room Mist
Spot Application	Anointing Oil

For more information, see Methods of Using Essential Oils on page xi.

Ravensara

Latin name: *Ravensara aromatica*

Country of origin: Madagascar

Part of the plant: Leaves

Extraction method: Steam distilled

Main biochemical components*: Limonene, alpha-terpinene, sabinene

Physical uses: Infections (bacterial, viral), respiratory congestion, colds, flu, bronchitis, sinusitis, coughs, laryngitis, indigestion, muscle fatigue, stiff joints, water retention, menstrual cramps, lymphatic support, immune support.

Skin care uses: Infections (bacterial, viral), small cuts, shingles, cold sores.

Psychological uses: Anxiety, stress, nervous fatigue, mild depression, fear.

Subtle uses: Supports desire for change. Releases fear.

Notes: Use Ravensara in a 1-5% dilution. Avoid during pregnancy and nursing.

* Chemical component percentages may vary. Essential 3 offers a *Certificate of Analysis* for review.

Methods of use:

After Shower	Bath
Bath, Foot	Chest Rub
Compress	Diffusion
Inhalation	Inhalation, Hot Water
Massage	Room Mist
Spot Application	Anointing Oil

For more information, see Methods of Using Essential Oils on page xi.

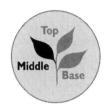

NOTES

Avoid during pregnancy and nursing
Highly anti-infectious
Immune stimulant
Respiratory antiviral

Which One?

Ravensara has a strong, clear, hint of sweet, herbaceous aroma. **Ravintsara** has a strong, refreshing, clear, camphoraceous aroma. Ravensara is higher in methyl chavicol and Ravintsara is higher in 1,8 cineole. They are both good for infections, respiratory congestion, muscle aches, and immune support. However, Ravintsara is considered to be a bit gentler.

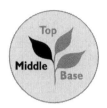

NOTES

Avoid during pregnancy
and nursing
Highly anti-infectious
Immune stimulant
Respiratory antiviral

Which One?

Ravensara has a strong, clear, hint of sweet, herbaceous aroma. **Ravintsara** has a strong, refreshing, clear, camphoraceous aroma. Ravensara is higher in methyl chavicol and Ravintsara is higher in 1,8 cineole. They are both good for infections, respiratory congestion, muscle aches, and immune support. However, Ravintsara is considered to be a bit gentler.

Ravintsara

Latin name: *Cinnamomum camphora cineoliferum*

Country of origin: Madagascar

Part of the plant: Leaves

Extraction method: Steam distilled

Main biochemical components*: 1,8-cineole, sabinene, beta-pinene

Physical uses: Infections (bacterial, viral), respiratory congestion, colds, flu, bronchitis, coughs, muscle aches, stiff joints, immune support, lymphatic support.

Skin care uses: Infections (bacterial, viral), small cuts and wounds, cold sores, shingles.

Psychological uses: Stress, anxiety, mild depression, mental fog.

Subtle uses: Supports desire for change. Releases fear.

Notes: Avoid Ravintsara during pregnancy and nursing.

* Chemical component percentages may vary. Essential 3 offers a *Certificate of Analysis* for review.

Methods of use:

After Shower	Bath
Bath, Foot	Chest Rub
Compress	Diffusion
Inhalation	Inhalation, Hot Water
Massage	Room Mist
Spot Application	Anointing Oil

For more information, see Methods of Using Essential Oils on page xi.

Rose

also known as Rose Otto

Latin name: *Rosa damascena*

Country of origin: E. Europe

Part of the plant: Flowers

Extraction method: Steam distilled (cohobation)

Main biochemical components*: Alkanes, alkenes, geraniol

Physical uses: Muscle spasms, inflammation, coughs, sore throats, feeling over-heated, nausea, headaches, infections, PMS, menopausal symptoms, circulatory tonic.

Skin care uses: Dry skin, mature skin, sensitive skin, irritated skin, inflammation, infections, eczema, wrinkles, skin tonic.

Psychological uses: Mild depression, stress, anxiety, irritability, tension, emotional coolness, low libido, sleeplessness, anger, fear.

Subtle uses: Brings in positive energy. Promotes love, compassion, hope, and patience. Promotes creativity and love of beauty. Helps to heal emotional wounds, especially grief.

Notes: Avoid Rose during first 4 months of pregnancy.

* Chemical component percentages may vary.
  Essential 3 offers a *Certificate of Analysis* for review.

Methods of use:

Add to Products	After Shower	Bath
Bath, Foot	Body Lotion	Body Oil
Chest Rub	Compress	Compress, Facial
Diffusion	Facial Oil	Inhalation
Inhalation, Hot Water	Massage	Perfume
Skin Mist	Spot Application	Anointing Oil

For more information, see Methods of Using Essential Oils on page xi.

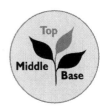

NOTES

Avoid during the first
4 months of pregnancy
Stress relief
Skin care
Aphrodisiac
Favorite perfume
Sleep aid
Also known as
Rose Otto

Which One?

The Roses have a deep, spicy-sweet, floral aroma. **E. Europe** has a bit softer, more refined aroma. It is steam distilled, producing a clear essential oil. **Morocco** has a bit stronger aroma. It is an absolute and is brownish-orange in color. Both are used for skin care, PMS, menopause, stress, as aphrodisiacs, and are favorite perfumes.

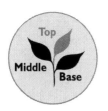

NOTES

Avoid during the first
4 months of pregnancy
Stress relief
Skin care
Aphrodisiac
Favorite perfume
Sleep aid

Rose (Morocco)
also known as Rose Absolute

Latin name: *Rosa centifolia*

Country of origin: Morocco

Part of the plant: Flowers

Extraction method: Absolute

Main biochemical components*: Geraniol, citronellol, nerol

Physical uses: Muscle spasms, inflammation, infections, coughs, sore throats, feeling over-heated, nausea, headaches, PMS, menopausal symptoms, circulatory tonic.

Skin care uses: Dry skin, mature skin, sensitive skin, irritated skin, inflammation, infections, eczema, wrinkles, skin tonic.

Psychological uses: Mild depression, stress, anxiety, irritability, tension, emotional coolness, low libido, sleeplessness, anger, fear.

Subtle uses: Brings in positive energy. Promotes love, compassion, hope, and patience. Promotes creativity and love of beauty. Helps to heal emotional wounds, especially grief.

Notes: Avoid Rose (Morocco) during first 4 months of pregnancy.

* Chemical component percentages may vary. Essential 3 offers a *Certificate of Analysis* for review.

Which One?
The Roses have a deep, spicy-sweet, floral aroma. **E. Europe** has a bit softer, more refined aroma. It is steam distilled, producing a clear essential oil. **Morocco** has a bit stronger aroma. It is an absolute and is brownish-orange in color. Both are used for skin care, PMS, menopause, stress, as aphrodisiacs, and are favorite perfumes.

Methods of use:

Add to Products	After Shower	Bath
Bath, Foot	Body Lotion	Body Oil
Chest Rub	Compress	Compress, Facial
Diffusion	Facial Oil	Inhalation
Inhalation, Hot Water	Massage	Perfume
Skin Mist	Spot Application	Anointing Oil

For more information, see Methods of Using Essential Oils on page xi.

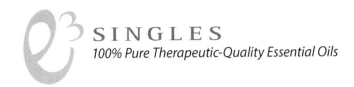
Rosemary, ct. cineole

Latin name: *Rosmarinus officinalis*

Country of origin: Morocco

Part of the plant: Leaves, twigs, flowers

Extraction method: Steam distilled

Main biochemical components*: Beta-thujone, camphor, 1,8 cineole

Physical uses: Respiratory congestion, infections, colds, flu, sinusitis, bronchitis, fatigue, poor circulation, muscle aches, stiff joints, general stimulant, immune support.

Skin care uses: Dandruff, scalp tonic, infections.

Psychological uses: Nervous exhaustion, chronic fatigue, mild depression, mental fatigue, mental fog.

Subtle uses: Clears energy blocks. Protects against negativity. Clears the mind. Promotes insight and understanding. Strengthens will power. Promotes self confidence. Helps to establish "healthy boundaries" in relationships. Inspires faith.

Notes: Use Rosemary, ct. cineole in a 1 to 5% dilution. Avoid during pregnancy and nursing. Avoid with high blood pressure.

* Chemical component percentages may vary. Essential 3 offers a *Certificate of Analysis* for review.

Methods of use:

After Shower	Bath
Bath, Foot	Chest Rub
Compress	Diffusion
Inhalation	Inhalation, Hot Water
Massage	Scalp Oil
Spot Application	Anointing Oil

For more information, see Methods of Using Essential Oils on page xi.

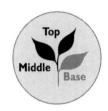

NOTES

Avoid w/high blood pressure

Avoid during pregnancy and nursing.

Stimulant

Improves concentration and focus

May not be compatible with homeopathics

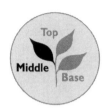

NOTES

"Bois de rose"

Stress relief

Skin care

Aphrodisiac

Rosewood

Latin name: *Aniba roseodora*

Country of origin: Brazil

Part of the plant: Wood

Extraction method: Steam distilled

Main biochemical components*: Linalol, alpha-cubebene, alpha-terpineol

Physical uses: Coughs, colds, flu, sore throats, nausea, muscle tonic, infections, immune support.

Skin care uses: Imbalanced oil production, dry skin, oily skin, devitalized skin, wrinkles, body odor, small wounds, infections, dermatitis, skin tonic.

Psychological uses: Anxiety, stress, tension, mood swings, mild depression, jet lag, emotional coolness, low libido.

Subtle uses: Brings in positive energy. Clears energy blocks. Promotes self-acceptance. Gently opens the mind and heart.

Notes: Rosewood is also known as "bois de rose."

* Chemical component percentages may vary. Essential 3 offers a *Certificate of Analysis* for review.

Methods of use:

Add to Products	After Shower
Bath	Bath, Foot
Body Lotion	Body Oil
Chest Rub	Compress
Compress, Facial	Diffusion
Facial Oil	Inhalation
Inhalation, Hot Water	Massage
Skin Mist	Spot Application
Anointing Oil	

For more information, see Methods of Using Essential Oils on page xi.

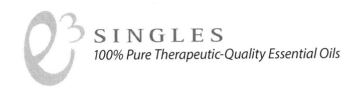

Sage

Latin name: *Salvia officinalis*

Country of origin: Greece

Part of the plant: Leaves

Extraction method: Steam distilled

Main biochemical components*: Beta-thujone, camphor, 1,8 cineole

Physical uses: Infections (bacterial, viral, fungal), coughs, colds, flu, sinusitis, bronchitis, muscle aches, stiff joints, water retention, immune support.

Skin care uses: Insect bites, small wounds, dermatitis, cold sores, oily skin, oily scalp, infections (bacterial, viral, fungal).

Psychological uses: Mild depression, mental exhaustion.

Subtle uses: Promotes courage, wisdom, emotional strength, and perseverance. Clears negativity.

Notes: Use Sage in a 1 to 5% dilution. Avoid during pregnancy and nursing.

* Chemical component percentages may vary. Essential 3 offers a *Certificate of Analysis* for review.

Methods of use:

After Shower	Bath, Foot
Chest Rub	Diffusion
Inhalation	Massage
Room Mist	Scalp Oil
Spot Application	Anointing Oil

For more information, see Methods of Using Essential Oils on page xi.

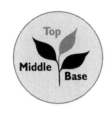

NOTES

Avoid during pregnancy and nursing

Air disinfectant

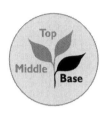

NOTES

Stress relief

Skin care

Meditation

Aphrodisiac

Favorite perfume

Sleep aid

Sandalwood (Mysore)

Latin name: *Santalum album*

Country of origin: India

Part of the plant: Heartwood

Extraction method: Steam distilled

Main biochemical components*: Cis-alpha-santalol, cis-beta-santalol, trans-alpha-bergamotol

Physical uses: Dry coughs, bronchitis, laryngitis, sore throats, respiratory congestion, inflammation, infections, muscle spasms, nerve pain, poor circulation, lymphatic support, immune support.

Skin care uses: Dry skin, mature skin, sensitive skin, rough skin, devitalized skin, oily skin, blemishes, eczema, itching, chapped skin, inflammation, infections, small wounds, skin tonic.

Psychological uses: Anxiety, tension, stress, sleeplessness, sense of isolation, emotional instability, low libido.

Subtle uses: Calms and comforts. Promotes the ability to trust and accept. Encourages meditative states. Promotes wisdom and a sense of peace.

Notes: Sandalwood (Mysore) is popular for meditation.

* Chemical component percentages may vary. Essential 3 offers a *Certificate of Analysis* for review.

Methods of use:

Add to Products	After Shower	Bath
Bath, Foot	Body Lotion	Body Oil
Chest Rub	Compress	Compress,
Facial	Diffusion	Facial Oil
Inhalation	Inhalation, Hot Water	
Massage	Perfume	Room Mist
Skin Mist	Spot Application	Anointing Oil

For more information, see Methods of Using Essential Oils on page xi.

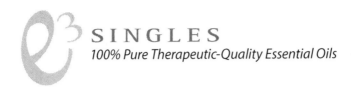

SINGLES
100% Pure Therapeutic-Quality Essential Oils

Spearmint

Latin name: *Mentha spicata*

Country of origin: USA

Part of the plant: Flowering tops (fresh)

Extraction method: Steam distilled

Main biochemical components*: Carvone, limonene, trans-carvylacetate

Physical uses: Respiratory congestion, bronchitis, sinusitis, colds, flu, fevers, infections, muscle aches, muscle spasms, stiff joints, indigestion, nausea, headaches, menstrual cramps.

Skin care uses: Oily skin, blemishes, congested skin, infections, body odor, itching, small wounds.

Psychological uses: Mental fatigue, mild depression.

Subtle uses: Clears energy blocks. Energizes, uplifts, and rejuvenates.

Notes: Use Spearmint in a 1 to 5% dilution. Avoid during pregnancy and nursing.

* Chemical component percentages may vary. Essential 3 offers a *Certificate of Analysis* for review.

Methods of use:

After Shower	Bath, Foot
Chest Rub	Compress
Diffusion	Inhalation
Inhalation, Hot Water	Massage
Room Mist	Skin Mist
Spot Application	Anointing Oil

For more information, see Methods of Using Essential Oils on page xi.

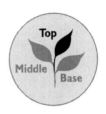

NOTES

Avoid during pregnancy and nursing

Gentle stimulant

Fatigue due to chemotherapy

Uplifting, fresh clean aroma

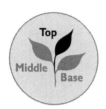

NOTES

Avoid use in sun

A gentle citrus

Stress relief

Uplifting, happy aroma

Tangerine

Latin name: *Citrus reticulata*

Country of origin: USA

Part of the plant: Rinds

Extraction method: Cold pressed

Main biochemical components*: Limonene, beta-phellandrene, gamma-terpinene

Physical uses: Muscle spasms, muscle aches, menstrual cramps, indigestion, constipation, digestive tonic, PMS, lymphatic support.

Skin care uses: Oily skin, blemishes, skin tonic.

Psychological uses: Stress, tension, anxiety, fear.

Subtle uses: Promotes joy and happiness.

Notes: Do not use Tangerine directly on the skin when you are going to be in the sun.

* Chemical component percentages may vary. Essential 3 offers a *Certificate of Analysis* for review.

Methods of use:

After Shower	Bath
Bath, Foot	Compress
Compress, Facial	Diffusion
Inhalation	Massage
Room Mist	Anointing Oil

For more information, see Methods of Using Essential Oils on page xi.

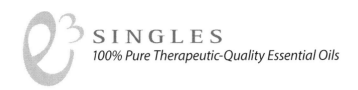

Tansy, Blue

Latin name: *Tanacetum annuum*

Country of origin: Morocco

Part of plant: Flowers

Extraction method: Steam distilled

Main biochemical components*: Sabinene, camphor, para-cymene, beta-pinene, chamazulene, alpha-phellandrene, dihydro-chamazulene isomer, myrcene, limonene

Physical uses: Inflamed muscles and joints, sprains, strains, fever, hypertension, arthritis, rheumatism, fibromyalgia, sciatica, nerve pain, headaches, indigestion, allergies.

Skin care uses: Inflammation, irritations, rashes, rosacea, itching, burns, sunburns, bruises.

Psychological uses: Nervous tension, depression especially with agitation, stress.

Subtle uses: Promotes inner peace and forgiveness.

Notes: Avoid during pregnancy and nursing.

* Chemical component percentages may vary. Essential 3 offers a *Certificate of Analysis* for review.

Methods of use:

Add to Product	After Shower
Bath	Bath, Foot
Body Lotion	Body Oil
Compress	Compress, Facial
Diffusion	Facial Oil
Inhalation	Massage
Skin Mist	Spot Application
Anointing Oil	

For more information, See Methods of Using Essential Oils on page xi.

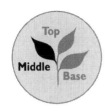

NOTES

Beneficial for allergies
Good anti-inflammatory
for use with burned,
damaged or
bruised skin

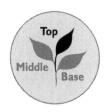

SINGLES
100% Pure Therapeutic-Quality Essential Oils

Top
Middle
Base

NOTES

Highly anti-infectious

Immune stimulant

May help protect skin

from radiation burns

Air disinfectant

Toenail fungus

Tea Tree

Latin name: *Melaleuca alternifolia*

Country of origin: Australia

Part of the plant: Leaves and twigs

Extraction method: Steam distilled

Main biochemical components*: Terpinen-4-ol, gamma-terpinene, alpha-terpinene

Physical uses: Infections (bacterial, viral, fungal), colds, flu, sinusitis, bronchitis, tonsillitis, poor circulation, sore throats, immune support.

Skin care uses: Infections (bacterial, viral, fungal), oily skin, blemishes, athlete's foot, nail fungus, cold sores, insect bites and stings, small wounds, dandruff, ringworm, warts.

Psychological uses: Nervous exhaustion, mild depression, mental fatigue.

Subtle uses: Energizes. Promotes confidence.

Notes: Tea Tree is known for its gentle yet powerful, full-spectrum, anti-infectious properties and its support for the immune system.

* Chemical component percentages may vary. Essential 3 offers a *Certificate of Analysis* for review.

Methods of use:

After Shower	Bath
Bath, Foot	Chest Rub
Compress, Facial	Diffusion
Inhalation	Inhalation, Hot Water
Massage	Room Mist
Scalp Oil	Spot Application
Anointing Oil	

For more information, see Methods of Using Essential Oils on page xi.

Thyme, ct. linalol

Latin name: *Thymus vulgaris*

Country of origin: France

Part of the plant: Leaves and flowering tops (dried or partially dried)

Extraction method: Steam distilled

Main biochemical components*: Terpinene, p-cymene, linalol, thymol

Physical uses: Infections (bacterial, viral, fungal), bronchitis, coughs, tonsillitis, muscle aches, muscle spasms, poor circulation, immune support.

Skin care uses: Infections (bacterial, viral, fungal), oily skin, blemishes, warts, small wounds, dandruff, scalp tonic.

Psychological uses: Nervous exhaustion, stress, mental fatigue, mental fog.

Subtle uses: Clears energy blocks. Promotes self-confidence. Focuses the mind.

Notes: Use Thyme, ct. linalol in a 1 to 5% dilution. Avoid during pregnancy and nursing.

* Chemical component percentages may vary. Essential 3 offers a *Certificate of Analysis* for review.

Methods of use:

After Shower	Bath, Foot
Chest Rub	Compress
Inhalation	Massage (specific area)
Room Mist	Scalp Oil
Spot Application	Anointing Oil

For more information, see Methods of Using Essential Oils on page xi.

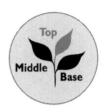

NOTES

Avoid during pregnancy and nursing
Highly anti-infectious
Immune stimulant
Blemishes

Which One?

Thyme, ct. linalol has a fresh, herbaceous, spicy, slightly sweet aroma. **Thyme, ct. thymol** has a sharp, woody-spicy, herbaceous, warm aroma. They are both highly anti-infectious and good immune stimulants. **Thymol** is stronger and more stimulating. Care must be taken with its use. **Linalol** is gentler and the best choice for use on the skin.

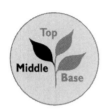

NOTES

Avoid during pregnancy

and nursing

Avoid w/high

blood pressure

Highly anti-infectious

Immune stimulant

Thyme, ct. thymol

Latin name: *Thymus vulgaris*

Country of origin: Spain

Part of the plant: Leaves and flowering tops (dried or partially dried)

Extraction method: Steam distilled

Main biochemical components*: Thymol, para-cymene, gamma-terpinene

Physical uses: Muscle spasms, muscle aches, stiff joints, colds, coughs, bronchitis, flu, respiratory congestion, infections (bacterial, viral, fungal), respiratory congestion, poor circulation, water retention, fatigue, immune support.

Skin care uses: Insect bites, dandruff, blemishes, infections (bacterial, viral, fungal), scalp tonic.

Psychological uses: Mental fatigue, mild depression, mental fog,

Subtle uses: Clears mental energy blocks. Promotes courage.

Notes: Use Thyme, ct. thymol in a 1 to 5% dilution. Avoid use during pregnancy. Avoid with high blood pressure.

* Chemical component percentages may vary.
  Essential 3 offers a *Certificate of Analysis* for review.

Which One?

Thyme, ct. linalol has a fresh, herbaceous, spicy, slightly sweet aroma. **Thyme, ct. thymol** has a sharp, woody-spicy, herbaceous, warm aroma. They are both highly anti-infectious and good immune stimulants. **Thymol** is stronger and more stimulating. Care must be taken with its use. **Linalol** is gentler and the best choice for use on the skin.

Methods of use:

Chest Rub	Compress
Inhalation	Massage (specific area)
Scalp Oil	Spot Application
Anointing Oil	

For more information, see Methods of Using Essential Oils on page xi.

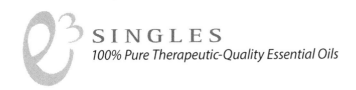

Valerian Root

Latin name: *Valeriana officinalis*

Country of origin: India

Part of the plant: Roots

Extraction method: Steam distilled

Main biochemical components*: Camphene, kessyl alcohol, valeranone

Physical uses: Muscle spasms, nerve pain, nervous indigestion.

Skin care uses: n/a

Psychological uses: Nervousness, tension, restlessness, sleeplessness.

Subtle uses: Comforts the heart.

Notes: Use Valerian Root in a 1 to 5% dilution. May be sensitizing. Avoid during pregnancy and nursing.

* Chemical component percentages may vary. Essential 3 offers a *Certificate of Analysis* for review.

Methods of use:

Compress	Inhalation
Massage	Spot Application
Anointing Oil	

For more information, see Methods of Using Essential Oils on page xi.

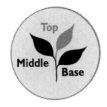

NOTES

May be sensitizing
Avoid during pregnancy
    and nursing
Calms high-anxiety
Sleep aid

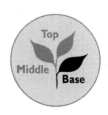

Top
Middle
Base

NOTES

Immune stimulant

Skin care

Meditation

Aphrodisiac

Grounding

Sleep aid

Deep, earthy aroma

Vetiver

Latin name: *Vetiveria zizanioides*

Country of origin: Haiti

Part of the plant: Roots (dried then soaked)

Extraction method: Hydro-diffused

Main biochemical components*: Vetiverol, alpha-vetivol, beta-vetivene

Physical uses: Muscle aches, stiff joints, poor circulation, infections, lymphatic support, immune support.

Skin care uses: Devitalized skin, dry skin, mature skin, rough skin, irritations, blemishes, infections, small wounds.

Psychological uses: Nervous tension, sleeplessness,
mild depression, mental exhaustion, emotional instability, low libido.

Subtle uses: Grounds, calms, and centers. Strengthens and protects. Promotes a deep sense of belonging. Promotes wisdom.

Notes: Vetiver is known for its deep, earthy, pervasive aroma.

* Chemical component percentages may vary.
   Essential 3 offers a *Certificate of Analysis* for review.

Methods of use:

After Shower	Bath
Bath, Foot	Body Lotion
Body Oil	Compress
Compress, Facial	Diffusion
Facial Oil	Inhalation
Massage	Skin Mist
Spot Application	Anointing Oil

For more information, see Methods of Using Essential Oils on page xi.

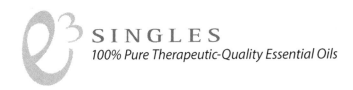
Wintergreen

Latin name: *Gaultheria procumbens*

Country of origin: China

Part of the plant: Leaves

Extraction method: Steam distilled

Main biochemical components*: Methyl salicylate

Physical uses: Muscle aches, muscle cramps, stiff joints, water retention, inflammation.

Skin care uses: Eczema, blemishes, inflammation, small wounds.

Psychological uses: Mental fog.

Subtle uses: Relaxes the logical mind. Dispels resistance to change. Promotes self-reflection.

Notes: Use Wintergreen highly diluted (1% or less)! May be sensitizing. Avoid during pregnancy and nursing. Allergies to methyl salicylate can be common, so a patch test is recommended before using Wintergreen. For short-term use.

* Chemical component percentages may vary. Essential 3 offers a *Certificate of Analysis* for review.

Methods of use:

Compress	Inhalation
Massage (specific area)	Spot Application
Anointing Oil	

For more information, see Methods of Using Essential Oils on page xi.

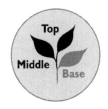

NOTES

Use highly diluted!
(1% or less)
May be sensitizing
Avoid during pregnancy
and nursing
Topical pain relief for
short-term use

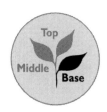

NOTES

May be sensitizing

Stress relief

Skin care

Sleep aid

Very sweet, floral aroma

Calming

Ylang Ylang, Extra

Latin name: *Cananga odorata*

Country of origin: Indonesia

Part of the plant: Flowers

Extraction method: Steam distilled

Main biochemical components*: Benzyl acetate, linalol, farnesol

Physical uses: Rapid breathing, tense breathing, general tension.

Skin care uses: Imbalanced oil production, dry skin, oily skin, mature skin, inflammation, itching, scalp tonic, skin tonic.

Psychological uses: Stress, anxiety, sleeplessness, nervous tension, mild depression, anger, shock, emotional coolness, low libido.

Subtle uses: Promotes a sense of peace. Dispels anger and fear. Promotes self-confidence and enthusiasm.

Notes: Use Ylang Ylang, Extra in a 1 to 5% dilution. May be sensitizing.

* Chemical component percentages may vary. Essential 3 offers a *Certificate of Analysis* for review.

Methods of use:

Add to Products	After Shower
Bath	Bath, Foot
Body Lotion	Body Oil
Compress	Compress, Facial
Diffusion	Facial Oil
Inhalation	Massage
Perfume	Room Mist
Skin Mist	Scalp Oil
Spot Application	Anointing Oil

For more information, see Methods of Using Essential Oils on page xi.

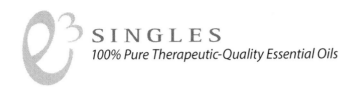

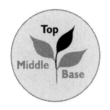

Yuzu

Latin name: *Citrus junos*

Country of origin: Japan

Part of the plant: Rinds

Extraction method: Cold pressed

Main biochemical components*: Limonene, myrcene, y-terpinene

Physical uses: Infections (bacterial, viral, fungal), stiff joints, colds, flu, lymphatic support, immune support.

Skin care uses: Infections (bacterial, viral, fungal), oily skin, body odor.

Psychological uses: Mild depression, anxiety, stress, tension, frustration, mental fog.

Subtle uses: Brings in positive energy. Clears energy blocks. Diminishes regret. Promotes self-confidence and focus.

Notes: Do not use Yuzu directly on the skin when you are going to be in the sun.

* Chemical component percentages may vary.
   Essential 3 offers a *Certificate of Analysis* for review.

Methods of use:

After Shower	Bath
Bath, Foot	Chest Rub
Diffusion	Inhalation
Massage	Room Mist
Spot Application	Anointing Oil

For more information, see Methods of Using Essential Oils on page xi.

NOTES

Avoid use in sun

Air freshener

Uplifting, citrus aroma

Stress relief

Japanese orange

Essential 3's Non-standard Singles, Synergy Blends, and Carrier Oils

To meet the needs of our varied customers, E3 stocks both *standard* and *non-standard* singles, synergy blends, and carrier oils. Our *standards* are profiled in detail in this booklet and on our website. They are sold in regular sizes, with our signature design label, and are appropriate for retail sales. Our *non-standards* are sold in the quantity requested with a simple, white label.

Following is a list of our current, non-standard singles, synergy blends, and carrier oils. Please contact us for pricing. If there is a non-standard you are looking for and do not see it here, let us know and we will check its availability.

SINGLES

EO	Latin name	Country of origin	Part of plant
African Sandalwood, Muhuhu	*Brachyleana hutchinsii*	Kenya	Heartwood
Allspice	*Pimenta dioica*	Jamaica	Fruit/berries
Amyris	*Amyris balsamifera*	Haiti	Wood
Anise Seed	*Pimpinella anisum*	Egypt	Seeds
Anise, Star	*Illicum vernum*	China	Fruit
Bay Oil (Rum)	*Pimenta racemusa*	Jamaica	Leaves
Birch, Sweet	*Betula lenta*	Canada	Bark
Cajeput	*Melaleuca cajuputi*	Australia	Leaves
Calamus	*Acorus calamus*	Nepal	Roots
Cassia	*Cinnamomum cassia*	China	Leaves/twigs
Catnip tops	*Nepeta cataria*	Canada	Flowering
Cedarwood, Western Red	*Thuja plicata*	Canada	Wood
Celery Seed	*Apium graveolens*	India	Seeds
Chili Pepper, CO2	*Capsicum frutescens*	India	Fruit
Choya Loban	*Boswellia serrata*	India	Resin
Cilantro	*Coriandrum sativum*	Egypt	Leaves
Cinnamon Bark	*Cinnamomum zeylanicum*	Indonesia	Bark
Cistus	*Cistus ladaniferus*	Spain	Leaves/Stalk
Cocoa, Absolute	*Theobroma cacao*	France	Beans
Coffee Oil	*Coffea arabica*	Venezuela	Beans
Combaya Petitgrain (Kaffir Lime)	*Citrus hystrix*	Madagascar	Leaves/twig
Cornmint	*Mentha arvensis*	India	Plant

EO	Latin name	Country of origin	Part of plant
Copaiba Balsam	Copaifera langsdorfii	South America	Balsam
Cumin	Cuminum cyminum	Egypt	Seeds
Cypress	Cupressus torulosa	Nepal	Wood
Davana	Artemisia pallens	India	Plant
Dill	Anethum graveolens	USA	Seeds
Elemi	Canarium luzonicum	Philippines	Resin
Erigeron (Fleabane)	Erigeron canadensis	USA	Plant
Fir Needle, Siberia	Abies siberica	Siberia	Needles
Fir Needle, White	Abies alba	Austria	Needles
Galangal Root	Alpine galangal	Indonesia	Root
Galbanum	Ferula galbaniflua	Iran	Resin
Gingerlily CO2	Hedychium spicatum	India	Rhizomes
Gingergrass var. Sofia	Cymbopogon martini	India	Grass
Helichrysum Gymnocephalum	Helichrysum gymnocephalum	Madagascar	Plant
Holy Basil	Ocimum santum	India	Leaves
Hyssop	Hyssopus decumbens	Spain	Plant
Lavandin Grosso tops	Lavandula x hybrida	France	Flowering
Ledum	Ledum groenlandicum	Canada	Plant
Lemon Oil, Green	Citrus limonum	Bolivia	Rinds
Lime (Distilled)	Citrus aurantifolia	Mexico	Rinds
Mandarin, Green	Citrus deliciosa	Italy	Rinds
Manuka	Leptospermum scoparium	New Zealand	Leaves
Massoia Bark	Cryptocaryo massoia	Indonesia	Bark
May Chang (Litsea Cubeba)	Litsea cubeba	China	Fruit
Melissa	Melissa officinalis	France	Flowering tops, leaves, stems
Mimosa, Absolute	Acacia decurrens	France	Flower
Myrtle, Lemon	Backhousia citriodora	Australia	Leaves
Myrtle, Red	Myrtus communis	Morocco	Leaves/Fruit
Oakmoss, Absolute	Evernia prunastri	France	Moss
Opoponax	Commiphora erythraea	Kenya	Resin
Orange, Bitter	Citrus aurantium	Brazil	Rinds

EO	Latin name	Country of origin	Part of plant
Orange, Blood	*Citrus sinensis*	Italy	Rinds
Orange, Dark	*Citrus sinensis*	Belize	Rinds
Parsley Seed	*Petroselinum sativum*	Indonesia	Seeds
Patchouli Light (Stainless Steel)	*Pogostemon cablin*	Indonesia	Leaves
Peach Artemisia	*Artemisia ludoviciana*	USA	Plant
Peru Balsam	*Myroxylon peruiferum*	El Salvador	Resin
Petitgrain (Lemon Leaf)	*Citrus limonum*	Spain	Leaves
Pink Pepper Tree	*Schinus molle*	Kenya	Fruit
Rosalina	*Melaleuca ericafolia*	Australia	Leaves
Sage, Spanish	*Salvia lavandulaefolia*	Spain	Leaves
Sea Buckthorn Berry Co_2	*Hippophae rhamnoides*	Lithuania	Fruit
Spikenard, Green	*Nardostachys jatamansi*	Nepal	Roots
Spruce	*Tsuga Canadensis*	Canada	Needles
Tangerine 5X	*Citrus reticulata*	USA	Rinds
Tarragon	*Artemisia dracunculus*	USA	Plant
Tobacco Absolute	*Nicotiana tobacum*	Bulgaria	Leaves
Turmeric	*Curcuma longa*	India	Rhizomes
Violet Leaf, Dilute	*Viola odorata*	Egypt	Leaves
Yarrow, Blue	*Achillea millefolium*	Bulgaria	Flower

SYNERGY BLENDS

Deep Healing	Helichrysum, Chamomile Roman, Chamomile German, Blue Tansy, Carrot Seed, Lavender (France, High Altitude)
Frankincense & Myrrh	Frankincense, Myrrh
Fruity Green Tea	Orange, Rosewood, Bay Laurel, Osmanthus Absolute, Rose Geranium
Grassy Tea	Clary Sage, Bay Laurel, Black Pepper, Fir Needle
Vanilla Blend	Opoponax, Vanilla Absolute, Benzoin, Myrrh

CARRIER OILS

Evening Primrose, CO2	*Oenothera biennis*	China	Seeds
Neem Seed, CO2	*Azadirachta indica*	India	Seeds

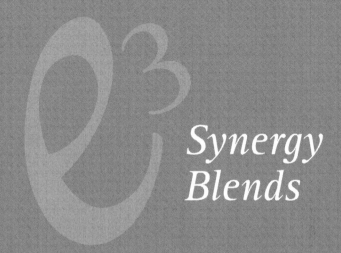

Synergy
Blends

THERAPEUTIC-QUALITY ESSENTIAL OILS
COMBINED ENHANCE
THEIR EFFECTIVENESS

"A perfumed bath and a scented massage every day is the way to good health."

— Hippocrates

"When the soul approaches the mysteries, when it tries to rally to the great spiritual principles, the perfumes are there."

— Marguerite Maury

℮³ SYNERGY BLENDS

Therapeutic-Quality Essential Oils
Combined to Enhance Their Effectiveness

A synergy is the interaction of two or more elements that create a combined effect that is greater than the sum of their individual effects.

Standard Synergy Blends

Essential 3 has created a collection of essential oil synergy blends for wellness and renewal. Each blend is created with therapeutic-quality essential oils, meticulously composed in perfect balance for a particular purpose and to achieve a specific result. Their names indicate their use and make selection easy.

Use the **Quick Reference Guide** and **Synergies for Systems of the Body** to help you find what you need. There is more information on each synergy, individually, in this section of the booklet.

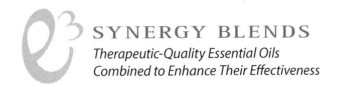

Therapeutic-Quality Essential Oils
Combined to Enhance Their Effectiveness

Quick Reference Guide

First Aid
Bruise & Scar, Migraine, Stress Relief, Nausea Relief, Nerve Calming Blend, Inflammation Blend

Stress Relief
Relax, Rebalance, Serenity, Stress Relief, Female Harmony, Sandalwood Blend, Adrenal Support, Nerve Calming Blend

Psychological Enhancement
Concentrate, Courageous, Habit Release, Mood Rescue, Relax, Rebalance, Revitalize, Female Harmony, Sandalwood Blend, Sensualize, Stress Relief, Male Harmony, Peace, Pick Me Up, Solace, Transition

Meditation / Spirituality
Meditate, Sandalwood Blend, Serenity

Aphrodisiac
Sensualize, Sandalwood Blend

Muscle / Joint Support
Muscle Soothe, Joint Relief, Massage Blend

Health Support
Cold & Sinus, Head Soothe, Lymphatic Support, Cardiovascular Support, Migraine, Nausea Relief, Protection, Sleeptime, Immune Blend, Digestion Blend, Adrenal Support, Endocrine Blend, Skin Care Blend, Nerve Calming Blend, Respiratory Blend, Urinary Blend

Women's Health
Female Harmony, Sensualize, Stress Relief, Nerve Calming Blend

Men's Health
Male Harmony, Sensualize, Stress Relief, Nerve Calming Blend

Air Quality
Antiseptic Blend, Purify, Protection

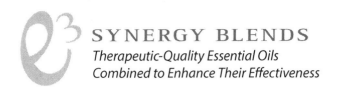

Synergy Blends for Systems of the Body

Circulatory (blood and lymph)
Lymphatic Support
Cardiovascular Support

Digestive
Nausea Relief
Digestion Blend

Endocrine
Adrenal Support
Endocrine Blend

Immune
Antiseptic Blend
Immune Blend
Protection

Integumentary
Bruise & Scar
Skin Care Blend

Musculoskeletal
Joint Relief
Muscle Soothe
Massage Blend

Nervous
Rebalance
Nerve Calming Blend

Reproductive
Sensualize
Female Harmony
Male Harmony

Respiratory
Breathe Easy
Cold & Sinus
Respiratory Blend

Urinary
Urinary Blend

SYNERGY BLENDS
Therapeutic-Quality Essential Oils
Combined to Enhance Their Effectiveness

NOTES

Chronic stress

After-illness depletion

Burn out

Adrenal Support

E3's Adrenal Support synergy blend is designed to stimulate circulation to the adrenal glands, revitalize, and relieve the stress that can lead to burn out (also known as adrenal exhaustion).

The following essential oils are in **Adrenal Support** (alphabetical order). The therapeutic uses that are listed for each essential oil are those that are relevant to the purpose of this particular blend.

Black Spruce: Fatigue, immune support, adrenal support, stress, anxiety, burn out.

Cedarwood, Atlas: Immune support, stress, tension, anxiety, emotional exhaustion.

Geranium: Poor circulation, immune support, general tonic, stress, anxiety, mild depression.

Peppermint: Sluggishness, immune support, nervous stress, mild depression, shock.

Pine Needle: Poor circulation, fatigue, immune support, adrenal support.

Vetiver: Poor circulation, immune support, nervous tension, mild depression, mental exhaustion.

For more information about the above, individual essential oils, please refer to the Singles section, beginning on page 1.

Methods of use:
Adrenal Support is best used intermittently.

Area massage: *Mix 6-15 drops of Adrenal Support in 1 tablespoon of fractionated coconut oil or fragrance-free, natural lotion. In the morning, massage the kidney area (on your back, just above the waist, towards the sides, beneath the rib cage).*

After Shower   Inhalation
Bath, Foot

For more information, see Methods of Using Essential Oils on page xi.

E³ SYNERGY BLENDS
Therapeutic-Quality Essential Oils
Combined to Enhance Their Effectiveness

Antiseptic Blend

NOTES

Bathroom air freshener

Hospital / hospice odors

Air disinfectant (especially

for sick rooms)

E3's Antiseptic synergy blend is designed to cleanse the air to lessen the possibility of infection while supporting the immune system.

The following essential oils are in **Antiseptic Blend** (alphabetical order). The therapeutic uses that are listed for each essential oil are those that are relevant to the purpose of this particular blend.

Clove: Infections, aches, wound healing.

Eucalyptus, Citriodora: Infections, inflammation, immune support.

Lavender: Infections, aches, inflammation, wound healing, skin tonic.

Lemon: Infections, itching, immune support, skin tonic.

Myrtle, Lemon: Infections, astringent.

Oregano: Infections, immune support.

Palmarosa: Infections, wound healing, skin tonic.

Rosemary, ct. cineole: Aches, infections, astringent, wound healing, skin tonic.

Sage: Infections, astringent, wound healing, skin tonic.

Thyme, ct. linalol: Infections, wound healing, skin tonic.

For more information about the above, individual essential oils, please refer to the Singles section, beginning on page 1.

Methods of use:
Diffusion   Room Mist

For more information, see Methods of Using Essential Oils on page xi.

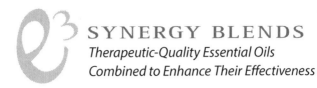

NOTES

Drop in shower or

steam room

Drop on tissue in

pillow case for sleeping

COPD: Rub on chest

Breathe Easy

E3's Breathe Easy synergy blend is designed to support comfortable, relaxed breathing.

The following essential oils are in **Breathe Easy Blend** (alphabetical order). The therapeutic uses that are listed for each essential oil are those that are relevant to the purpose of this particular blend.

Eucalyptus, Citriodora: Tense breathing, immune support, anxiety, stress, nervous tension, mild depression.

Eucalyptus, Radiata: Respiratory congestion, immune support, mild depression, apathy.

Eucalyptus, Smithii: Respiratory congestion, immune support, mild depression, apathy.

Peppermint: Respiratory congestion, muscle spasms, mental fatigue, mental fog, nervous stress, mild depression.

For more information about the above, individual essential oils, please refer to the Singles section, beginning on page 1.

Methods of use:

Chest Rub	Compress
Diffusion	Inhalation
Inhalation, Hot Water	

For more information, see Methods of Using Essential Oils on page xi.

Bruise & Scar

NOTES

Apply to bruise immediately

Apply to wound after it has closed or stitches are removed

E3's Bruise & Scar synergy blend is designed to lessen the healing time of bruises, ease discomfort and inflammation, and to minimize the appearance of a newly forming scar.

A bruise is an injury to the skin caused by trauma that breaks blood vessels and causes blood to leak into surrounding tissue. A scar is the result of the body's natural healing process to repair a wound. Scar tissue is different than the tissue it replaces.

The following essential oils are in **Bruise & Scar** (alphabetical order). The therapeutic uses that are listed for each essential oil are those that are relevant to the purpose of this particular blend.

Cypress: Wound healing, bruising, poor circulation, astringent, skin tonic.

Frankincense: Wound healing, inflammation, minor bleeding, astringent, skin tonic.

Helichrysum: Inflammation, wound healing, bruising, astringent. (The best known essential oil for bruises.)

Lavender: Aches, wound healing, itching, minor bleeding, skin tonic.

Petitgrain: Inflammation, skin tonic.

Rose: Inflammation, wound healing, minor bleeding, astringent, skin tonic.

Rosewood: Aches, wound healing, skin tonic.

For more information about the above, individual essential oils, please refer to the Singles section, beginning on page 1.

Methods of use:
Compress   Spot application
Massage *(Gently massaging a scar will help keep skin pliable and reduce tissue build-up, minimizing its appearance.)*

For more information, see Methods of Using Essential Oils on page xi.

SYNERGY BLENDS
Therapeutic-Quality Essential Oils
Combined to Enhance Their Effectiveness

NOTES

Long drives or flights

Sedentary lifestyle

Lengthy sitting

Cardiovascular Support

E3's Cardiovascular Support synergy blend is designed to support cardiovascular circulation, relax tense muscles and breathing, and relieve nervous tension.

The following essential oils are in **Cardiovascular Support** (alphabetical order). The therapeutic uses that are listed for each essential oil are those that are relevant to the purpose of this particular blend.

Cypress: Poor circulation, water retention, muscle cramps and spasms, nervous tension.

Geranium: Poor circulation, circulatory congestion, general tonic, stress, anxiety.

Grapefruit, Red: Poor circulation, water retention, nervous exhaustion.

Marjoram, Sweet: Muscle spasms, tense breathing, stress, tension.

Orange, Sweet: Poor circulation, water retention, nervous tension.

Rosemary, ct. cineole: Poor circulation, nervous exhaustion, chronic fatigue.

For more information about the above, individual essential oils, please refer to the Singles section, beginning on page 1.

Methods of use:

After Shower	Bath
Bath, Foot	Body Lotion
Body Oil	Compress
Massage	

For more information, see Methods of Using Essential Oils on page xi.

E3 SYNERGY BLENDS
Therapeutic-Quality Essential Oils
Combined to Enhance Their Effectiveness

Child Harmony

E3's Child Harmony synergy blend is designed to soothe and calm children when they are upset, cranky, or over-tired, and when they need to calm down and relax for bedtime. It can also be used to appease the inner child of adults.

The following essential oils are in **Child Harmony** (alphabetical order). The therapeutic uses that are listed for each essential oil are those that are relevant to the purpose of this particular blend.

Chamomile, Roman: Irritability, restlessness, anxiety, tension, anger, stress, impatience, shock, hyperactivity.

Dill: Anxiety, overwhelm, chaos, upset tummy.

Fennel, Sweet: Emotional weakness, fear, anxiety, upset tummy.

Lavender: Exhaustion, imbalance, irritability, restlessness, anxiety, anger, tension, stress.

Mandarin, Red: Restlessness, melancholy, anxiety.

For more information about the above, individual essential oils, please refer to the Singles section, beginning on page 1.

Methods of use:
(Child Harmony is for children over the age of 3. See side column for age-appropriate dilution information intended for this synergy blend.)

Massage: *Mix 1-10 drops in 1 oz fragrance-free, natural lotion and gently massage the child's back. If tummy is upset, gently massage abdomen in the direction/flow of the colon.*

Diffusion: *Use 2-5 drops.*

Bath: *Mix 1-4 drops in ½ cup of whole milk or 1 teaspoon of fractionated coconut oil. Set aside. Fill the bathtub with warm water. Immerse child. Add essential oil mixture and stir the water.*

"Magic Wand": *Roll and twist a paper towel. Put 2-3 drops on the end and allow the child to wave it and breathe in the aroma.*

Cloth Toy: *Put 1-2 drops on a favorite cloth toy.*

For more information, see Methods of Using Essential Oils on page xi.

NOTES

Over tired

Over stimulated

Travel anxiety

School / study anxiety

Dilution for Kids
Baths
(dilute in 2 tsp of carrier)
3-5 years .....1-2 drops
   and use ½ of this
   amount in bath
6-10 years ...1-3 drops
11 + years ...1-4 drops

Massage
(dilute in 1 oz of carrier)
3-4 years .....1-5 drops
5-7 years ......3-6 drops
8-12 years ...5-9 drops
12 + years ...5-10 drops

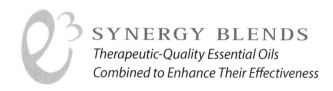

SYNERGY BLENDS
Therapeutic-Quality Essential Oils
Combined to Enhance Their Effectiveness

Drop on tissue in

pillowcase for sleeping

Drop in shower or

steam room

Foot massage

Cold & Sinus

E3's Cold & Sinus synergy blend is designed to soothe the symptoms of colds and allergies, while supporting the immune system and easing discomfort.

The following essential oils are in **Cold & Sinus** (alphabetical order). The therapeutic uses that are listed for each essential oil are those that are relevant to the purpose of this particular blend.

Cajeput: Infections, respiratory congestion, fevers.

Eucalyptus, Globulus: Infections, respiratory congestion, sore throats, fevers, immune support.

Lavender: Infections, muscle aches, respiratory congestion, lymphatic support.

Peppermint: Infections, respiratory congestion, fevers, muscle aches, lymphatic support, immune support.

Tea Tree: Infections, respiratory congestion, immune support.

For more information about the above, individual essential oils, please refer to the Singles section, beginning on page 1.

Methods of use:

After Shower	Bath, Foot
Chest Rub	Diffusion
Inhalation	Inhalation, Hot Water
Massage	Room Mist

For more information, see Methods of Using Essential Oils on page xi.

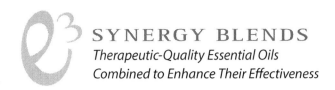
Concentrate

E3's Concentrate synergy blend is designed to promote mental alertness, concentration, and focus.

The following essential oils are in **Concentrate** (alphabetical order). The therapeutic uses that are listed for each essential oil are those that are relevant to the purpose of this particular blend.

Frankincense: Restless mind.

Orange, Sweet: Mental fatigue, mild depression.

Peppermint: Physical and mental fatigue, mental fog, mild depression.

Rosemary, ct. cineole: Physical and mental fatigue, mental fog, mild depression.

For more information about the above, individual essential oils, please refer to the Singles section, beginning on page 1.

Methods of use:

After Shower	Bath, Foot
Diffusion	Inhalation
Massage	Room Mist

For more information, see Methods of Using Essential Oils on page xi.

NOTES

For studying

For taking a test

For mental focus

Afternoon meetings

Office productivity

Courageous

E3's Courageous synergy blend is designed to calm, relax, and settle the mind and body, while promoting **mental clarity and fortitude.**

The following essential oils are in **Courageous** (alphabetical order). The therapeutic uses that are listed for each essential oil are those that are relevant to the purpose of this particular blend.

Black Spruce: Mental fog, mental spaciness.

Blue Tansy: Tension, anxiety, stress.

Frankincense: Tension, shallow breathing, rapid breathing, stress, emotional instability.

Rosewood: Emotional imbalance, emotional instability, tension, anxiety, stress.

For more information about the above, individual essential oils, please refer to the Singles section, beginning on page 1.

Methods of use:

After Shower	Anointing Oil
Bath, Foot	Body Lotion
Body Oil	Diffusion
Inhalation	Massage
Perfume	Room Mist

For more information, see Methods of Using Essential Oils on page xi.

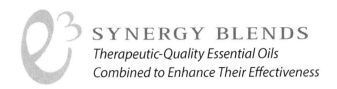

SYNERGY BLENDS
*Therapeutic-Quality Essential Oils
Combined to Enhance Their Effectiveness*

Digestion Blend

E3's Digestion synergy blend is designed to ease indigestion and lift the spirits to support good digestion.

The following essential oils are in **Digestion Blend** (alphabetical order). The therapeutic uses that are listed for each essential oil are those that are relevant to the purpose of this particular blend.

Black Pepper: Indigestion, sluggish digestion.

Cardamom: Indigestion, nausea, heartburn, stomach ache, anxiety, mild depression.

Mandarin, Red: Indigestion, stress, anxiety, tension, mild depression, restlessness.

Nutmeg: Indigestion, nausea.

Rosemary, ct. cineole: Sluggish digestion, mild depression.

Spearmint: Indigestion, nausea, mild depression.

For more information about the above, individual essential oils, please refer to the Singles section, beginning on page 1.

Methods of use:
Bath, Foot
Compress
Inhalation
Massage (stomach and esophagus areas)

For more information, see Methods of Using Essential Oils on page xi.

NOTES

Too full

Weak digestion

Indigestion

e3 SYNERGY BLENDS
Therapeutic-Quality Essential Oils
Combined to Enhance Their Effectiveness

PMS

Menopause

Andropause

Feeling out-of-balance

Endocrine Blend

E3's Endocrine synergy blend is designed to support good circulation, promote deep breathing for oxygenation, to ease stress and to help harmonize the body.

The following essential oils are in **Endocrine Blend** (alphabetical order). The therapeutic uses that are listed for each essential oil are those that are relevant to the purpose of this particular blend.

Frankincense: Tense breathing, shallow breathing, rapid breathing, anxiety, stress, nervous tension.

Geranium: Poor circulation, circulatory congestion, mood swings, general tonic.

Orange, Sweet: Poor circulation, lymphatic support, nervous tension, mild depression, worry.

Patchouli: Tense breathing, rapid breathing, nervous exhaustion, stress, mild depression.

Sandalwood: Poor circulation, lymphatic support, anxiety, tension, stress, sleeplessness, emotional instability.

For more information about the above, individual essential oils, please refer to the Singles section, beginning on page 1.

Methods of use:

After Shower	Bath
Bath, Foot	Body Lotion
Body Oil	Inhalation
Massage	

For more information, see Methods of Using Essential Oils on page xi.

Female Harmony

E3's Female Harmony synergy blend is designed to ease the discomfort and imbalances of PMS, peri-menopause, and menopause, and to promote a sense of well-being.

The following essential oils are in **Female Harmony** (alphabetical order). The therapeutic uses that are listed for each essential oil are those that are relevant to the purpose of this particular blend.

Chamomile, Roman: Muscle aches, menstrual cramps, upset stomach, muscle tension, headaches, irregular cycle, nervous tension, mild depression, emotional discomfort, worry, irritability, anxiety, sleeplessness, stress.

Clary Sage: Menstrual cramps, muscle aches, muscle tension, irregular cycle, imbalance, nervous tension, mild depression, anxiety, stress, sleeplessness, emotional discomfort, lack of sense of well-being.

Geranium: Muscle aches, poor circulation, imbalance, mild depression, mood swings.

Palmarosa: Poor circulation, fatigue, irritability, stress, mild depression, mental fog.

Rose: Menstrual cramps, irregular cycle, muscle tension, mild depression, emotional imbalance, emotional discomfort, headaches, anxiety, stress, low libido, sleeplessness.

Sandalwood: Menstrual cramps, muscle tension, poor circulation, emotional discomfort, anxiety, stress, sleeplessness, low libido.

For more information about the above, individual essential oils, please refer to the Singles section, beginning on page 1.

Methods of use:

After Shower	Anointing Oil	Bath
Bath, Foot	Body Lotion	Body Oil
Compress	Diffusion	Facial Oil
Inhalation	Massage	Skin Mist

For more information, see Methods of Using Essential Oils on page xi.

NOTES column (handwritten):
PMS
Menopause
Menstrual cramps
Feeling out-of-balance

NOTES

Supports change

Habit Release

E3's Habit Release synergy blend is designed to support the intentional change of routine behavior (habits).

The following essential oils are in **Habit Release** (alphabetical order). The therapeutic uses that are listed for each essential oil are those that are relevant to the purpose of this particular blend.

Benzoin: Emotional weakness, anxiety, tension, stress, mild depression.

Clary Sage: Nervous tension, mild depression, anxiety, stress, sleeplessness, emotional discomfort, lack of sense of well-being.

Frankincense: Restless mind, anxiety, tension, stress.

For more information about the above, individual essential oils, please refer to the Singles section, beginning on page 1.

Methods of use:

After Shower	Anointing Oil
Bath	Bath, Foot
Body Lotion	Body Oil
Compress	Diffusion
Inhalation	Massage
Room Mist	

For more information, see Methods of Using Essential Oils on page xi.

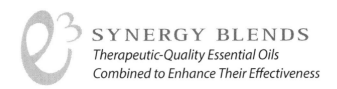

Head Soothe

E3's Head Soothe synergy blend is designed to soothe physical and emotional tension—relax tight muscles, calm anxiety, ease stress, and uplift the spirit.

The following essential oils are in **Head Soothe** (alphabetical order). The therapeutic uses that are listed for each essential oil are those that are relevant to the purpose of this particular blend.

Chamomile, Roman: Muscle aches, muscle spasms, muscle tension, mild depression, over-sensitivity, emotional discomfort, worry, shock, tension, anxiety, stress.

Geranium: Muscle aches, poor circulation, mild depression, imbalance, mood swings.

Lavender: Muscle aches, muscle spasms, sinus congestion, inflammation, mild depression, emotional discomfort, tension, anxiety, stress.

Peppermint: Muscle aches, muscle spasms, headaches, inflammation, nerve pain, sinus congestion, feeling over-heated, mild depression, anger.

For more information about the above, individual essential oils, please refer to the Singles section, beginning on page 1.

Methods of use:

After Shower	Bath, Foot
Compress	Inhalation
Massage	Spot Application

For more information, see Methods of Using Essential Oils on page xi.

NOTES

Massage back of neck and shoulders

Stress relief

Muscle tension

Mild depression

NOTES

Airplane travel

When in crowds

Cold and flu season

Mild depression

Immune Blend

E3's Immune synergy blend is designed to support the immune and lymphatic systems.

The following essential oils are in **Immune Blend** (alphabetical order). The therapeutic uses that are listed for each essential oil are those that are relevant to the purpose of this particular blend.

Black Spruce: Fatigue, sluggishness, infections, stress, immune support, adrenal support.

Cistus: Infections, lymphatic support.

Lemon: Infections, poor circulation, mild depression, immune support.

Niaouli: Infections, fatigue, sluggishness, immune support.

Oregano: Infections, sluggishness, immune support.

Plai: Infections, poor circulation, stress.

Thyme, ct. linalol: Infections, poor circulation, stress, immune support.

Ylang Ylang, Extra: Physical tension, tense breathing, nervous tension, mild depression, stress.

For more information about the above, individual essential oils, please refer to the Singles section, beginning on page 1.

Methods of use:

After Shower	Bath, Foot
Diffusion	Inhalation
Massage	

For more information, see Methods of Using Essential Oils on page xi.

Inflammation Blend

E3's Inflammation synergy blend is designed to calm and soothe inflammation as well as support the lymphatic and immune systems.

The following essential oils are in **Inflammation Blend** (alphabetical order). The therapeutic uses that are listed for each essential oil are those that are relevant to the purpose of this particular blend.

Chamomile, German: Inflammation, headaches, nerve pain.

Helichrysum: Inflammation, poor circulation, nerve pain, immune support.

Lavender: Lymphatic support, inflammation, infections.

Peppermint: Nerve pain, aches, infections, lymphatic support.

Tea Tree: Infections, immune support.

Wintergreen: Inflammation, aches.

For more information about the above, individual essential oils, please refer to the Singles section, beginning on page 1.

Methods of use:
Compress (use with cool water)
Massage (gentle)
Spot Application

For more information, see Methods of Using Essential Oils on page xi.

NOTES

Strained ankles

Strained muscles

NOTES

Minor strains

After workouts

Stiff / sore joints

Jogging aches

Joint Relief

E3's Joint Relief synergy blend is designed to warm and soothe to promote comfort and mobility. Use whenever needed, especially before or after exercising, gardening, or other physical activity.

The following essential oils are in **Joint Relief** (alphabetical order). The therapeutic uses that are listed for each essential oil are those that are relevant to the purpose of this particular blend.

Eucalyptus, Globulus: Aches, stiff joints. (Exceptionally penetrating.)

Juniperberry: Spasms, cramps, stiff joints, poor circulation.

Lavender: Aches, inflammation, spasms, cramps.

Marjoram, Sweet: Aches, spasms, cramps, stiff joints.

Pine Needle: Inflammation, stiff joints, poor circulation. (Exceptionally penetrating.)

For more information about the above, individual essential oils, please refer to the Singles section, beginning on page 1.

Methods of use:

After Shower	Bath
Bath, Foot	Compress
Massage	Spot Application

For more information, see Methods of Using Essential Oils on page xi.

Lymphatic Support

E3's Lymphatic Support synergy blend is designed to support the lymphatic system and its processes of fighting infections, detoxifying, and working with the immune system. (The body has two circulatory systems, the cardiovascular and the lymphatic.)

The following essential oils are in **Lymphatic Support** (alphabetical order). The therapeutic uses that are listed for each essential oil are those that are relevant to the purpose of this particular blend.

Bay Laurel: Infections, poor circulation, lymphatic support, immune support.

Cypress: Infections, poor circulation, lymphatic support.

Geranium: Infections, circulatory congestion, poor circulation, lymphatic support, immune support.

Ginger: Infections, poor circulation.

Lemon: Infections, poor circulation, immune support.

Rosemary, ct. cineole: Infections, poor circulation, circulatory congestion, immune support.

Yuzu: Infections, lymphatic support.

For more information about the above, individual essential oils, please refer to the Singles section, beginning on page 1.

Methods of use:

After Shower	Body Lotion
Body Oil	Massage

For more information, see Methods of Using Essential Oils on page xi.

NOTES

When dieting

For detoxing

Recovering from illness

Male Harmony

E3's Male Harmony synergy blend is designed to ease the discomfort and imbalances of andropause issues and promote a sense of well-being.

The following essential oils are in **Male Harmony** (alphabetical order). The therapeutic uses that are listed for each essential oil are those that are relevant to the purpose of this particular blend.

Bergamot, FCF: Immune support, mild depression, stress, anxiety, nervousness, mood swings, apathy.

Cedarwood, Atlas: Poor lymphatic circulation, immune support, stress, tension, anxiety, emotional exhaustion, emotional instability.

Frankincense: Tense breathing, shallow breathing, rapid breathing, immune support, anxiety, stress, nervous tension, fear, restless mind.

Lavender: Tense breathing, lymphatic support, stress, nervous tension, anxiety, nervous exhaustion, mood swings, anger, sleeplessness.

Pine Needle: Poor circulation, fatigue, adrenal support, immune support, mental fatigue, nervous exhaustion.

Tea Tree: Poor circulation, immune support, nervous exhaustion, mild depression, mental fatigue.

For more information about the above, individual essential oils, please refer to the Singles section, beginning on page 1.

Methods of use:

After Shower	Bath
Bath, Foot	Body Lotion
Body Oil	Diffusion
Inhalation	Massage

For more information, see Methods of Using Essential Oils on page xi.

Massage Blend

NOTES

E3's Massage synergy blend is designed to help relax and soothe overworked muscles and emotional tension.

The following essential oils are in **Massage Blend** (alphabetical order). The therapeutic uses that are listed for each essential oil are those that are relevant to the purpose of this particular blend.

Eucalyptus, Globulus: Muscle aches, stiff joints, fatigue, poor circulation.

Fir Needle, Douglas: Muscle aches, poor circulation, mild depression, tension.

Lavender: Muscle aches, muscle tension, muscle spasms, cramps, anxiety, tension, nervous exhaustion, mood swings, stress.

Niaouli: Muscle aches, stiff joints, fatigue, poor circulation.

Peppermint: Muscle aches, muscle spasms, cramps, fatigue, sciatica, stress, mild depression, lymphatic support.

Rosemary, ct. cineole: Muscle aches, stiff joints, fatigue, nervous exhaustion, mild depression.

Tea Tree: Fatigue, poor circulation, inflammation, nervous exhaustion.

For more information about the above, individual essential oils, please refer to the Singles section, beginning on page 1.

Methods of use:

After Shower	Bath, Foot
Compress	Massage
Spot Application	

For more information, see Methods of Using Essential Oils on page xi.

Notes (handwritten):
Muscle tension
Poor circulation
Feeling out-of-balance

E³ SYNERGY BLENDS
*Therapeutic-Quality Essential Oils
Combined to Enhance Their Effectiveness*

NOTES

With yoga

For mental calm

Stress relief

Feeling unstable

Meditate

E3's Meditate synergy blend is designed to relax the body, quiet the mind, and uplift the spirit, while creating an intentional "sacred space" to enhance the meditation experience.

The following essential oils are in **Mediate** (alphabetical order). The therapeutic uses that are listed for each essential oil are those that are relevant to the purpose of this particular blend.

Bergamot, FCF: Mild depression, emotional imbalance, tension, stress, apathy.

Cedarwood, Atlas: Tension, stress, restless mind.

Frankincense: Tension, stress, shallow breathing, rapid breathing, restless mind.

Patchouli: Mild depression, tension, stress, emotional imbalance, emotional instability.

Sandalwood: Emotional discomfort, restless mind, stress, sense of isolation.

For more information about the above, individual essential oils, please refer to the Singles section, beginning on page 1.

Methods of use:

After Shower	Anointing Oil
Bath	Bath, Foot
Body Oil	Body Lotion
Diffusion	Inhalation
Massage	Perfume
Room Mist	

For more information, see Methods of Using Essential Oils on page xi.

SYNERGY BLENDS
Therapeutic-Quality Essential Oils
Combined to Enhance Their Effectiveness

Migraine

E3's Migraine synergy blend is designed to help relieve the symptoms of migraine headaches.

The following essential oils are in **Migraine** (alphabetical order). The therapeutic uses that are listed for each essential oil are those that are relevant to the purpose of this particular blend.

Basil, ct. linalol: Aches, muscle spasms, nervous tension, poor circulation.

Cardamom: Aches, muscle spasms, poor circulation, tension.

Chamomile, Roman: Aches, inflammation, muscle spasms, tension, stress, worry, anxiety, anger, fear.

Grapefruit, Red: Poor circulation, mild depression, nervous exhaustion.

Juniperberry: Poor circulation, mild depression, anxiety.

Lemongrass: Aches, poor circulation, vascular tension, mild depression, stress, anxiety, nervous exhaustion.

Marjoram, Sweet: Aches, muscle spasms, vascular tension, nerve pain, stress, mild depression, irritability, trauma.

Peppermint: Aches, muscle spasms, nerve pain, stress, anger, mild depression, shock.

Wintergreen: Aches, muscle spasms, inflammation.

For more information about the above, individual essential oils, please refer to the Singles section, beginning on page 1.

Methods of use:

After Shower	Bath, Foot
Compress	Diffusion
Inhalation	Massage
Spot Application	

For more information, see Methods of Using Essential Oils on page xi.

Massage back of neck and shoulders
Mild depression

E3 SYNERGY BLEND'S
Therapeutic-Quality Essential Oils
Combined to Enhance Their Effectiveness

Great "ahhh" bath

Feeling out-of-balance

Stress relief

Mood swings

Mood Rescue

E3's Mood Rescue synergy blend is designed to gently uplift, balance, and refresh the emotions, while promoting a sense of well-being.

The following essential oils are in **Mood Rescue** (alphabetical order). The therapeutic uses that are listed for each essential oil are those that are relevant to the purpose of this particular blend.

Bergamot, FCF: Mild depression, mood swings, stress, anxiety, tension, apathy.

Clary Sage: Stress, tension, mild depression, fear, panic, lack of sense of well-being.

Frankincense: Tense breathing, rapid breathing, shallow breathing, anxiety, stress, nervous tension, restless mind.

Lime: Mild depression, apathy, anxiety, mental fatigue.

For more information about the above, individual essential oils, please refer to the Singles section, beginning on page 1.

Methods of use:

After Shower	Bath
Bath, Foot	Diffusion
Inhalation	Perfume
Room Mist	

For more information, see Methods of Using Essential Oils on page xi.

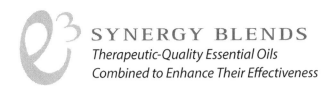

SYNERGY BLENDS
Therapeutic-Quality Essential Oils
Combined to Enhance Their Effectiveness

Muscle Soothe

NOTES

E3's Muscle Soothe synergy blend is designed to soothe overworked muscles due to physical activities such as sports, gardening, or exercising.

The following essential oils are in **Muscle Soothe** (alphabetical order). The therapeutic uses that are listed for each essential oil are those that are relevant to the purpose of this particular blend.

Fennel, Sweet: Muscle spasms, lymphatic support.

Lavender: Muscle aches, muscle tension, muscle spasms, cramps, anxiety, tension, nervous exhaustion, mood swings, stress.

Lemon: Poor circulation.

Lemongrass: Muscle aches, muscle fatigue, stiff joints, poor circulation, lymphatic support.

Peppermint: Muscle aches, muscle spasms, cramps, fatigue, sciatica, stress, mild depression, lymphatic support.

Rosemary, ct. cineole: Muscle aches, stiff joints, fatigue, nervous exhaustion, mild depression.

For more information about the above, individual essential oils, please refer to the Singles section, beginning on page 1.

Methods of use:

After Shower	Bath, Foot
Compress	Massage
Spot Application	

For more information, see Methods of Using Essential Oils on page xi.

Massage specific areas
Pre work out
Post work-out

Indigestion

Motion sickness

Nervous stomach

Nausea Relief

E3's Nausea Relief synergy blend is designed to calm a queasy, unsettled stomach.

The following essential oils are in **Nausea Relief** (alphabetical order). The therapeutic uses that are listed for each essential oil are those that are relevant to the purpose of this particular blend.

Chamomile, Roman: Stomach ache, nervousness, stress, anxiety, tension.

Elemi: Weak constitution.

Ginger: Indigestion, nausea.

Peppermint: Poor digestion, indigestion, stomach ache, nausea, motion sickness, nervous stress.

For more information about the above, individual essential oils, please refer to the Singles section, beginning on page 1.

Methods of use:

After Shower	Bath, Foot
Compress	Diffusion
Inhalation	Massage
Room Mist	Spot Application

For more information, see Methods of Using Essential Oils on page xi.

Nerve Calming Blend

E3's Nerve Calming synergy blend is designed to relax breathing, relax the muscles, calm the mind, and uplift the spirits to promote a sense of composure and peace.

The following essential oils are in **Nerve Calming Blend** (alphabetical order). The therapeutic uses that are listed for each essential oil are those that are relevant to the purpose of this particular blend.

Bergamot, FCF: Immune support, mild depression, stress, anxiety, nervousness, mood swings, apathy.

Chamomile, Roman: Muscle aches, headaches, PMS, nerve pain, stress, tension, anxiety, anger, fear, sleeplessness, worry, shock, impatience.

Lavender: Tense breathing, muscle aches, headaches, stress, nervous tension, anxiety, nervous exhaustion, mood swings, anger, sleeplessness.

Lemongrass: Muscle aches, jet lag, immune support, stress, anxiety, nervous exhaustion, mild depression.

Marjoram, Sweet: Muscle aches, PMS, tense breathing, nerve pain, headaches, stress, tension, irritability, trauma, mild depression, restlessness, sleeplessness.

Petitgrain: Tense breathing, immune support, stress, anxiety, tension, nervous exhaustion, panic, sleeplessness, mild depression.

For more information about the above, individual essential oils, please refer to the Singles section, beginning on page 1.

Methods of use:

After Shower	Bath
Bath, Foot	Body Oil
Body Lotion	Diffusion
Inhalation	Massage
Perfume	Room Mist

For more information, see Methods of Using Essential Oils on page xi.

NOTES

Chronic stress

Anxiety

Shock

Mood swings

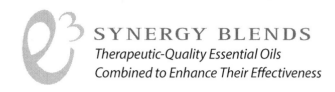

SYNERGY BLENDS
Therapeutic-Quality Essential Oils
Combined to Enhance Their Effectiveness

NOTES

Massage therapist's room

mist before session

A drop on tissue, inhale

to calm anxiety

Peace

E3's Peace synergy blend is designed to create a sense of inner calm and stillness.

The following essential oils are in **Peace** (alphabetical order). The therapeutic uses that are listed for each essential oil are those that are relevant to the purpose of this particular blend.

Lavender: Tense breathing, muscle spasms, muscle aches, headaches, itching, stress, nervous tension, anxiety, nervous exhaustion, mood swings, anger, sleeplessness.

Orange, Sweet: Nervous tension, mild depression, worry, mental fatigue.

Patchouli: Tense breathing, rapid breathing, nervous exhaustion, stress, mood swings, mild depression.

Tangerine: Muscle spasms, muscle aches, stress, tension, anxiety, fear.

Ylang Ylang Extra: Rapid breathing, tense breathing, general tension, stress, anxiety, sleeplessness, nervous tension, mild depression, anger, shock.

For more information about the above, individual essential oils, please refer to the Singles section, beginning on page 1.

Methods of use:

After Shower.	Bath
Bath, Foot	Body Lotion
Body Oil	Chest Rub
Diffusion	Inhalation
Massage	Room Mist

For more information, see Methods of Using Essential Oils on page xi.

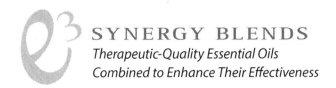

Pick Me Up

E3's Pick Me Up synergy blend is designed to uplift the spirits and reduce fatigue.

The following essential oils are in **Pick Me Up** (alphabetical order). The therapeutic uses that are listed for each essential oil are those that are relevant to the purpose of this particular blend.

Bergamot, FCF: Immune support, mild depression, stress, anxiety, nervousness, mood swings, apathy.

Lavender: Stress, tense breathing, nervous tension, anxiety, nervous exhaustion, mood swings, anger.

Lemon: Immune support, mental fog, mental clarity, mild depression.

Lemongrass: Stress, anxiety, nervous exhaustion, mental fatigue, mental fog, mild depression.

Melissa: Rapid breathing, anxiety, mild depression, tension, fear, crisis, shock, anger.

Orange, Sweet: Nervous tension, mild depression, worry, mental fatigue.

Peppermint: Mental fatigue, mental fog, anger, nervous stress, mild depression, shock.

For more information about the above, individual essential oils, please refer to the Singles section, beginning on page 1.

Methods or use:

Bath, Foot	Chest Rub
Diffusion	Inhalation
Massage	Room Mist

For more information, see Methods of Using Essential Oils on page xi.

NOTES

Uplifting

Mood enhancer

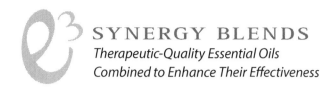

NOTES

Wipe door knobs

Wipe phones

Mist countertops

Airplane travel

When in crowds

Air filters

Protection

E3's Protection synergy blend is designed to provide defense for infections and support the immune system.

The following essential oils are in **Protection** (alphabetical order). The therapeutic uses that are listed for each essential oil are those that are relevant to the purpose of this particular blend.

Cinnamon Leaf: Infections, poor circulation, immune support.

Clove Bud: Infections, poor circulation.

Eucalyptus, Globulus: Infections, immune support.

Lemon: Infections, poor circulation, immune support.

Rosemary, ct. cineole: Infections, fatigue, immune support.

For more information about the above, individual essential oils, please refer to the Singles section, beginning on page 1.

Methods of use:

After Shower	Bath, Foot
Body Lotion	Body Oil
Chest Rub	Diffusion
Inhalation	Massage
Room Mist	

For more information, see Methods of Using Essential Oils on page xi.

Purify

E3's Purify synergy blend is designed to cleanse and deodorize. It is used to support the body's natural, detoxifying processes as well as to cleanse the air.

The following essential oils are in **Purify** (alphabetical order). The therapeutic uses that are listed for each essential oil are those that are relevant to the purpose of this particular blend.

Bergamot, FCF: Infections, deodorant, immune support.

Geranium: Infections, poor circulation, circulatory congestion, lymphatic support, immune support, general tonic, skin tonic.

Juniperberry: Poor circulation, infections, lymphatic support, astringent, immune support.

Lavender, Spike: Infections, immune support.

Pine Needle: Infections, poor circulation, water retention, immune support.

For more information about the above, individual essential oils, please refer to the Singles section, beginning on page 1.

Methods of use:

After Shower	Bath
Bath, Foot	Body Oil
Body Lotion	Diffusion
Massage	Room Mist
Skin Mist	

For more information, see Methods of Using Essential Oils on page xi.

NOTES

Hospital / hospice odors

Detox bath

Immune support

Air disinfectant

NOTES

Feeling out-of-balance

Mood swings

Feeling "ungrounded"

_____

_____

_____

_____

_____

_____

_____

_____

_____

_____

_____

_____

_____

_____

_____

_____

Rebalance

E3's Rebalance synergy blend is designed to balance and stabilize the emotions, promoting optimism, strength, and resilience.

The following essential oils are in **Rebalance** (alphabetical order). The therapeutic uses that are listed for each essential oil are those that are relevant to the purpose of this particular blend.

Bergamot, FCF: Mild depression, mood swings, apathy, stress, anxiety.

Cedarwood, Atlas: Exhaustion, stress, tension, anxiety, emotional instability

Geranium: Mild depression, moods swings, stress, anxiety.

Mandarin, Red: Stress, anxiety, tension, mild depression, restlessness.

Sandalwood: Anxiety, tension, stress, sense of isolation, sleeplessness, emotional instability.

Vetiver: Nervous tension, sleeplessness, mild depression, mental exhaustion, emotional instability.

For more information about the above, individual essential oils, please refer to the Singles section, beginning on page 1.

Methods of use:

After Shower	Bath
Bath, Foot	Body Lotion
Body Oil	Diffusion
Inhalation	Massage
Perfume	Room Mist
Skin Mist	

For more information, see Methods of Using Essential Oils on page xi.

Relax

E3's Relax synergy blend is designed to calm and relax the body, mind, and spirit. It is useful during the day or to promote a deep, restorative sleep at night.

The following essential oils are in **Relax** (alphabetical order). The therapeutic uses that are listed for each essential oil are those that are relevant to the purpose of this particular blend.

Geranium: Mild depression, moods swings, stress, anxiety.

Lavender: Stress, nervous tension, anxiety, nervous exhaustion, moods swings, anger, sleeplessness.

Marjoram, Sweet: Stress, tension, irritability, trauma, mild depression, restlessness, sleeplessness.

Vetiver: Nervous tension, sleeplessness, mild depression, mental exhaustion, emotional instability.

For more information about the above, individual essential oils, please refer to the Singles section, beginning on page 1.

Methods of use:

After Shower	Bath
Bath, Foot	Body Lotion
Body Oil	Diffusion
Inhalation	Massage
Perfume	Room Mist
Skin Mist	

For more information, see Methods of Using Essential Oils on page xi.

NOTES

Stress relief

Irritability

Massage therapist's room mist before session

Sleep aid

NOTES

Cold and flu

Immune support

Congestion

Respiratory Blend

E3's Respiratory synergy blend is designed to relax breathing, ease congestion, lessen the possibility of infection, and support the immune system.

The following essential oils are in **Respiratory Blend** (alphabetical order). The therapeutic uses that are listed for each essential oil are those that are relevant to the purpose of this particular blend.

Black Spruce: Respiratory congestion, poor circulation, immune support.

Eucalyptus, Citriodora: Infections, immune support.

Eucalyptus, Globulus: Respiratory congestion, infections, colds, flu, bronchitis, sore throats, fevers, immune support.

Eucalyptus, Radiata: Respiratory congestion, infections, colds, flu, bronchitis, sore throats, fevers, immune support.

Lavender: Respiratory congestion, bronchitis, laryngitis, colds, flu, tense breathing, infections.

Marjoram, Sweet: Sinusitis, bronchitis, coughing spasms, tense breathing.

Myrtle, Lemon: Respiratory congestion, bronchitis, sinusitis, infections.

Peppermint: Respiratory congestion, sinusitis, coughs, infections, immune support.

For more information about the above, individual essential oils, please refer to the Singles section, beginning on page 1.

Methods of use:

Chest Rub	Compress
Diffusion	Inhalation
Inhalation, Hot Water	

For more information, see Methods of Using Essential Oils on page xi.

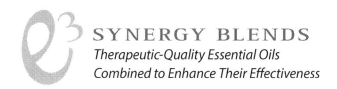

SYNERGY BLENDS
Therapeutic-Quality Essential Oils
Combined to Enhance Their Effectiveness

Revitalize

E3's Revitalize synergy blend is designed to uplift and rejuvenate the psyche. It also makes a mood-enhancing, air freshener.

The following essential oils are in **Revitalize** (alphabetical order). The therapeutic uses that are listed for each essential oil are those that are relevant to the purpose of this particular blend.

Bergamot, FCF: Mild depression, mood swings, apathy, stress, anxiety.

Grapefruit, Red: Poor circulation, muscle fatigue.

Mandarin, Red: Mild depression, stress, anxiety, tension, restlessness, sleeplessness.

Orange, Sweet: Poor circulation, nervous tension, mild depression, worry, mental fatigue.

For more information about the above, individual essential oils, please refer to the Singles section, beginning on page 1.

Methods of use:

After Shower	Anointing Oil
Bath, Foot	Diffusion
Inhalation	Perfume
Room Mist	

For more information, see Methods of Using Essential Oils on page xi.

NOTES

Uplifting mood enhancer

Mild depression

Apathy

Worry

NOTES

Great for blends

Skin care

Popular earthy aroma

for men and women

Meditation

Sandalwood Blend

E3's Sandalwood synergy blend is designed to offer the qualities and wonderful, earthy aroma of sandalwood at a lesser cost than pure Sandalwood from Mysore, India.

The following essential oils are in **Sandalwood Blend** (alphabetical order). The therapeutic uses that are listed for each essential oil are those that are relevant to the purpose of this particular blend.

Sandalwood (Australia, Eastern/Western): Dry coughs, sore throats, laryngitis, respiratory congestion, inflammation, muscle spasms, nerve pain, poor circulation, lymphatic support, immune support, dry skin, mature skin, sensitive skin, rough skin, devitalized skin, blemishes, eczema, itching, small wounds, anxiety, stress, tension, emotional instability, sleeplessness, sense of isolation, low libido.

Sandalwood (Mysore): Dry coughs, sore throats, laryngitis, respiratory congestion, inflammation, muscle spasms, nerve pain, poor circulation, lymphatic support, immune support, dry skin, mature skin, sensitive skin, rough skin, devitalized skin, blemishes, eczema, itching, small wounds, anxiety, stress, tension, emotional instability, sleeplessness, sense of isolation, low libido.

Sandalwood (Africa) also known as Muhuhu: Inflammation, muscle spasms, small wounds, aches, anxiety, stress, tension, emotional instability, sleeplessness, low libido.

For more information about the above, individual essential oils, please refer to the Singles section, beginning on page 1.

Methods of use:

After Shower	Bath	Bath, Foot
Body Lotion	Body Oil	Chest Rub
Compress	Compress, Facial	Diffusion
Facial Oil	Inhalation	Perfume
Inhalation, Hot Water	Massage	Skin Mist
Spot Application	*For more information, see*	

Methods of Using Essential Oils on page xi.

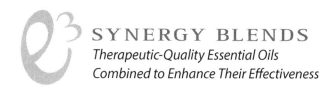

Sensualize

NOTES

E3's Sensualize synergy blend is designed to relax, build confidence, promote joy, and encourage emotional warmth and closeness.

The following essential oils are in **Sensualize** (alphabetical order). The therapeutic uses that are listed for each essential oil are those that are relevant to the purpose of this particular blend.

Orange, Sweet: Poor circulation, nervous tension, mild depression, worry, mental fatigue.

Patchouli: Nervous exhaustion, stress, lethargy, mood swings, mild depression, low libido.

Ylang Ylang, Extra: Nervous tension, stress, anxiety, mild depression, emotional coolness, low libido.

For more information about the above, individual essential oils, please refer to the Singles section, beginning on page 1.

Methods of use:

After Shower	Anointing Oil
Bath	Bath, Foot
Body Lotion	Body Oil
Diffusion	Inhalation
Massage	Perfume
Room Mist	Skin Mist

For more information, see Methods of Using Essential Oils on page xi.

Notes (handwritten):
Linen mist
Mood enhancer
Romantic body lotion
Romantic bath
Creative endeavors

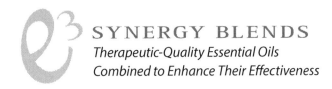

SYNERGY BLENDS
*Therapeutic-Quality Essential Oils
Combined to Enhance Their Effectiveness*

NOTES

Grief

Blends well with Meditate

Stress relief

Feeling "ungrounded"

Mild depression

Serenity

E3's Serenity synergy blend is designed to calm, comfort, and stabilize, while enveloping the psyche in tranquility and peace.

The following essential oils are in **Serenity** (alphabetical order). The therapeutic uses that are listed for each essential oil are those that are relevant to the purpose of this particular blend.

Bergamot, FCF: Mild depression, mood swings, apathy, stress, anxiety.

Cedarwood, USA: Stress, tension, anxiety, emotional tension.

Frankincense: Anxiety, stress, nervous tension, fear, restless mind.

Lime: Mild depression, apathy, anxiety, mental fatigue.

Rose: Mild depression, stress, anxiety, irritability, tension, emotional coolness, sleeplessness, anger, fear.

Vetiver: Nervous tension, tense breathing, rapid breathing, sleeplessness, mild depression, mental exhaustion, emotional instability.

Ylang Ylang, Extra: Stress, anxiety, sleeplessness, nervous tension, mild depression, anger, shock, emotional coolness.

For more information about the above, individual essential oils, please refer to the Singles section, beginning on page 1.

Methods of use:

After Shower	Bath
Bath, Foot	Body Lotion
Body Oil	Diffusion
Inhalation	Massage
Perfume	Room Mist

For more information, see Methods of Using Essential Oils on page xi.

Skin Care Blend

E3's Skin Care synergy blend is designed to soothe, condition, protect, and rejuvenate the skin.

The following essential oils are in **Skin Care Blend** (alphabetical order). The therapeutic uses that are listed for each essential oil are those that are relevant to the purpose of this particular blend.

Carrot Seed: Dry skin, sun-damaged skin, mature skin, devitalized skin, eczema, scars, calluses, rashes, burns, couperose, rosacea, skin tonic.

Frankincense: Wrinkles, dry skin, mature skin, scars, inflammation, small wounds, infections, skin tonic.

Lavender: Imbalanced oil production, small wounds, bruises, burns, sunburn insect bites and stings, infections, irritations, itching, blemishes, eczema, skin tonic.

Orange, Sweet: Dull, oily, puffy, rough or dry skin, wrinkles, poor circulation, infections, skin tonic.

Rosewood: Imbalanced oil production, dry skin, oily skin, devitalized skin, wrinkles, small wounds, infections, dermatitis, skin tonic.

Sandalwood: Dry skin, mature skin, sensitive skin, rough skin, devitalized skin, oily skin, blemishes, eczema, itching, chapped skin, inflammation, infection, small wounds, skin tonic.

Ylang Ylang, Extra: Imbalanced oil production, dry skin, oily skin, mature skin, inflammation, itching, skin tonic.

For more information about the above, individual essential oils, please refer to the Singles section, beginning on page 1.

Methods of use:

After Shower	Bath	Bath, Foot
Body Lotion	Body Oil	Compress
Compress, Facial	Facial Oil	Massage
Skin Mist	Spot Application	

For more information, see Methods of Using Essential Oils on page xi.

Notes (handwritten):
Conditions and beautifies
All skin types
Anti-aging

e³ SYNERGY BLENDS
Therapeutic-Quality Essential Oils
Combined to Enhance Their Effectiveness

NOTES

Diffuse before bedtime

Drop on tissue in

pillowcase

To "unwind"

Stress relief

Sleeptime

E3's Sleeptime synergy blend is designed to relax and comfort before bedtime to encourage a deeply restful and rejuvenating sleep.

The following essential oils are in **Sleeptime** (alphabetical order). The therapeutic uses that are listed for each essential oil are those that are relevant to the purpose of this particular blend.

Chamomile, Roman: Sleeplessness, stress, tension, anxiety, anger, fear, worry, shock, impatience.

Lavender: Sleeplessness, stress nervous tension, anxiety, nervous exhaustion, mood swings, anger.

Mandarin, Red: Sleeplessness, mild depression, stress, anxiety, tension, restlessness.

Sandalwood: Sleeplessness, anxiety, tension, stress, sense of isolation, emotional instability.

For more information about the above, individual essential oils, please refer to the Singles section, beginning on page 1.

Methods of use:

After Shower	Bath
Bath, Foot	Body Lotion
Body Oil	Chest Rub
Compress	Diffusion
Inhalation	Massage
Room Mist	

For more information, see Methods of Using Essential Oils on page xi.

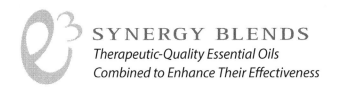

SYNERGY BLENDS
Therapeutic-Quality Essential Oils
Combined to Enhance Their Effectiveness

Solace

E3's Solace synergy blend is designed to provide gentle comfort and support when needed.

The following essential oils are in **Solace** (alphabetical order). The therapeutic uses that are listed for each essential oil are those that are relevant to the purpose of this particular blend.

Geranium: Immune support, stress, anxiety, mood swings, mild depression.

Helichrysum: Muscle aches, immune support, mild depression, nervous exhaustion, shock.

Peppermint: Respiratory congestion, muscle spasms, mental fatigue, mental fog, nervous stress, mild depression.

Wintergreen: Muscle aches, muscle cramps, mental fog.

Ylang Ylang Extra: Rapid breathing, tense breathing, general tension, stress, anxiety, sleeplessness, nervous tension, mild depression, anger, shock.

For more information about the above, individual essential oils, please refer to the Singles section, beginning on page 1.

Methods of use:

Bath, Foot	Chest Rub
Diffusion	Inhalation
Room Mist	Spot Application

For more information, see Methods of Using Essential Oils on page xi.

NOTES

Comforts

Soothes

Drop on a tissue,

inhale aroma

E3 SYNERGY BLENDS
Therapeutic-Quality Essential Oils
Combined to Enhance Their Effectiveness

De-stress coming

home from work

Shock

Mild depression

Stress Relief

E3's Stress Relief synergy blend is designed to calm the mind and relax the body to promote a sense of comfort, stability, and well-being.

The following essential oils are in **Stress Relief** (alphabetical order). The therapeutic uses that are listed for each essential oil are those that are relevant to the purpose of this particular blend.

Bergamot, FCF: Mild depression, mood swings, apathy, stress, anxiety.

Clary Sage: Stress, tension, anxiety, lack of sense of well-being, mild depression, fear, panic.

Geranium: Mild depression, moods swings, stress, anxiety.

Lavender: Stress, nervous tension, anxiety, nervous exhaustion, moods swings, anger, sleeplessness.

Mandarin, Red: Mild depression, stress, anxiety, tension, sleeplessness, restlessness.

For more information about the above, individual essential oils, please refer to the Singles section, beginning on page 1.

Methods of use:

After Shower	Bath
Bath, Foot	Body Lotion
Body Oil	Diffusion
Inhalation	Massage
Perfume	Room Mist

For more information, see Methods of Using Essential Oils on page xi.

Transition

E3's Transition synergy blend is designed to promote ease during times of change.

The following essential oils are in **Transition** (alphabetical order). The therapeutic uses that are listed for each essential oil are those that are relevant to the purpose of this particular blend.

Bergamot, FCF: Mild depression, stress, anxiety, nervousness, mood swings, apathy.

Black Spruce: Stress, anxiety, mental fog.

Frankincense: Tense breathing, rapid breathing, anxiety, stress, nervous tension, fear, restless mind.

Geranium: Stress, anxiety, mood swings, mild depression.

Hyssop, Decumbens: Tense breathing, anxiety, tension, stress, mild depression, mental fog, inability to concentrate.

Melissa: Rapid breathing, anxiety, mild depression, tension, crisis, fear, shock, anger.

Myrrh: Anxiety, tension, emotional coolness, apathy.

Rose: Mild depression, stress, anxiety, irritability, tension, emotional coolness, sleeplessness, anger, fear.

Rosewood: Anxiety, stress, tension, mood swings, mild depression, emotional coolness.

Sandalwood: Anxiety, tension, stress, sleeplessness, sense of isolation, emotional instability.

For more information about the above, individual essential oils, please refer to the Singles section, beginning on page 1.

Methods of use:

After Shower	Bath
Bath, Foot	Body Lotion
Body Oil	Diffusion
Inhalation	Massage
Room Mist	

For more information, see Methods of Using Essential Oils on page xi.

NOTES

*Drop on a tissue,
inhale aroma
Promotes calm during
times of change*

NOTES

UTI

Drop on pad for
bladder spasms

Urinary Blend

E3's Urinary synergy blend is designed to gently soothe and help prevent infections.

The following essential oils are in **Urinary Blend** (alphabetical order). The therapeutic uses that are listed for each essential oil are those that are relevant to the purpose of this particular blend.

Bergamot: Infections, immune support.

Chamomile, Roman: Inflammation, infections, irritations, itching, allergic reactions.

Geranium: Infections, poor circulation, general tonic, immune support.

Lavender: Infections, inflammation, irritations, itching, lymphatic support.

Tea Tree: Infections, poor circulation, immune support.

For more information about the above, individual essential oils, please refer to the Singles section, beginning on page 1.

Methods of use:

After Shower (lower back, abdomen)

Sitz Bath: *Fill the bathtub with enough warm (not hot) water to cover the hips, sitting, with knees up. Mix 6 drops of Urinary Blend in one tablespoon of fractionated coconut oil and stir well, then add this mixture to the bath water and agitate the water to mix well. Sit in the water for about fifteen minutes.*

Compress (lower back, abdomen)

Massage (lower back, abdomen)

For more information, see Methods of Using Essential Oils on page xi.

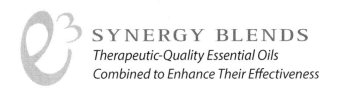

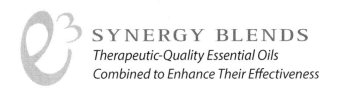SYNERGY BLENDS
Therapeutic-Quality Essential Oils
Combined to Enhance Their Effectiveness

Hospice Synergy Blends

E3's Hospice Blends, a collection of essential oil synergy blends, were developed by a clinical aromatherapist with over fifteen years of experience in hospice settings. **They were designed to accompany and complement the profound, personal journeys of those coming to the end-of-life and those family and friends who are present for it.** These blends have been sensitively created to provide comfort and support for all those involved; whether at home, the hospital, or a nursing home. Their aromas help facilitate beneficial responses such as connection, relaxation, and a sense of peace.

You will find the following 5 blends listed in both the Standard Synergy Blends section of this booklet as well as here in the Hospice Synergy Blends section. Although these blends were originally created for use in the hospice setting their benefits extend beyond the hospice community; health care practitioners and individuals alike, use these blends to support the health and well-being of their clients, themselves and their families.

SYNERGY BLENDS
Therapeutic-Quality Essential Oils
Combined to Enhance Their Effectiveness

Hospice Breathe Easy

E3's Hospice Breathe Easy is designed to support comfortable, relaxed breathing. It was developed by a clinical aromatherapist with over fifteen years of experience in hospice settings.

The following essential oils are in **Hospice Breathe Easy** (alphabetical order). The therapeutic uses that are listed for each essential oil are those that are relevant to the purpose of this particular blend. In a hospice setting, the emotional and spiritual effects of essential oils may become especially important, and for this reason, the subtle aromatherapy uses are also listed.

Eucalyptus, Citriodora: Tense breathing, immune support, anxiety, stress, nervous tension, mild depression.
Subtle aromatherapy: Clears and balances, uplifts, revitalizes, promotes letting go, comforts, promotes a sense of freedom.

Eucalyptus, Radiata: Respiratory congestion, immune support, mild depression, apathy.
Subtle aromatherapy: Clears negativity, balances, centers, inspires.

Eucalyptus, Smithii: Respiratory congestion, immune support, mild depression, apathy.
Subtle aromatherapy: Clears negativity, balances, centers.

Peppermint: Respiratory congestion, muscle spasms, mental fatigue, mental fog, nervous stress, mild depression.
Subtle aromatherapy: Promotes clarity in communication, inspires, awakens, encourages insights, refreshes, promotes self-acceptance.

For more information about the above, individual essential oils, please refer to the Singles section, beginning on page 1.

Methods of use:
Intention: When using essential oils in subtle aromatherapy, they are used with intention. This simply means that you state, silently or aloud, the purpose for which you are using the essential oils and visualize the desired results.

Inhalation   Gentle massage   Anointing

For more information, see Methods of Using Essential Oils on page xi.

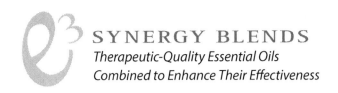

Therapeutic-Quality Essential Oils
Combined to Enhance Their Effectiveness

NOTES

COPD: Rub on chest.

Anxiety attack: Mix 4 drops Breathe Easy, 1 drop Lavender, and 1 drop Frankincense with 1 teaspoon of fractionated coconut oil or fragrance-free, natural lotion. Apply to upper back.

Bed baths: In 1/2 gallon of water, mix 3 drops Breathe Easy with 1 tablespoon Epsom salts. (Do not wash face or genital area.)

SYNERGY BLENDS
Therapeutic-Quality Essential Oils
Combined to Enhance Their Effectiveness

Hospice Peace

E3's Hospice Peace is designed to create a sense of peace. It was developed by a clinical aromatherapist with over fifteen years of experience in hospice settings.

The following essential oils are in **Hospice Peace** (alphabetical order). The therapeutic uses that are listed for each essential oil are those that are relevant to the purpose of this particular blend. In a hospice setting, the emotional and spiritual effects of essential oils may become especially important, and for this reason, the subtle aromatherapy uses are also listed.

Lavender: Tense breathing, muscle spasms, muscle aches, headaches, itching, stress, nervous tension, anxiety, nervous exhaustion, mood swings, anger, sleeplessness.
Subtle aromatherapy: Promotes inner peace, balances, calms, brings in positive energy, promotes a sense of acceptance, comforts, relaxes, promotes compassion.

Orange, Sweet: Nervous tension, mild depression, worry, mental fatigue.
Subtle aromatherapy: Brings in positive energy, promotes joy and happiness, balances, revitalizes, lightens the heart.

Patchouli: Tense breathing, rapid breathing, nervous exhaustion, stress, mood swings, mild depression.
Subtle aromatherapy: Grounds, strengthens, relaxes the intellectual mind, soothes, restores.

Tangerine: Muscle spasms, muscle aches, stress, tension, anxiety, fear.
Subtle aromatherapy: Promotes joy and happiness, refreshes, revitalizes, promotes a sense of peace, soothes.

Ylang Ylang Extra: Rapid breathing, tense breathing, general tension, stress, anxiety, sleeplessness, nervous tension, mild depression, anger, shock.
Subtle aromatherapy: Uplifts, promotes a sense of well-being, calms, soothes, promotes joy and enthusiasm.

For more information about the above, individual essential oils, please refer to the Singles section, beginning on page 1.

Methods of use:
Intention: When using essential oils in subtle aromatherapy, they are used with intention. This simply means that you state, silently or aloud, the purpose for which you are using the essential oils and visualize the desired results.

Inhalation   Gentle massage   Anointing

For more information, see Methods of Using Essential Oils on page xi.

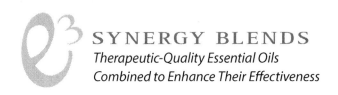

NOTES

Terminal agitation

Mix 12 drops Peace in 1 ounce of fractionated coconut oil or fragrance-free, natural lotion. Massage behind ears. If person can't move, massage hands, each finger, arms, feet, and legs.

Diffuse in room for family.

Hospice Pick Me Up

E3's Hospice Pick Me Up synergy blend is designed to uplift the spirits and reduce fatigue.

The following essential oils are in Pick Me Up (alphabetical order). The therapeutic uses that are listed for each essential oil are those that are relevant to the purpose of this particular blend.

Bergamot, FCF: Immune support, mild depression, stress, anxiety, nervousness, mood swings, apathy.
Subtle aromatherapy: Brings in positive energy, eases grief, promotes self-love, opens the heart and allows love to radiate, promotes joy, balances, encourages, promotes confidence.

Lavender: Stress, tense breathing, nervous tension, anxiety, nervous exhaustion, mood swings, anger.
Subtle aromatherapy: Promotes inner peace, balances, calms, brings in positive energy, promotes a sense of acceptance, comforts, relaxes, promotes compassion.

Lemon: Immune support, mental fog, mental clarity, mild depression.
Subtle aromatherapy: Clears energy blocks, clears emotional confusion, promotes mental clarity and objectivity, revitalizes, promotes joy, awakens.

Lemongrass: Stress, anxiety, nervous exhaustion, mental fatigue, mental fog, mild depression.
Subtle aromatherapy: Clears enegy block and dispels negativity.

Melissa: Rapid breathing, anxiety, mild depression, tension, fear, crisis, shock, anger.
Subtle aromatherapy: Uplifts, promotes understanding and acceptance, helps to ease grief, promotes a sense of peace, happiness and cheerfulness.

Orange, Sweet: Nervous tension, mild depression, worry, mental fatigue.
Subtle aromatherapy: Brings in positive energy, promotes joy and happiness, balances, revitalizes, lightens the heart.

Peppermint: Mental fatigue, mental fog, anger, nervous stress, mild depression, shock.
Subtle aromatherapy: Promotes clarity in communication, inspires, awakens, encourages insights, refreshes, promotes self-acceptance.

For more information about the above, individual essential oils, please refer to the Singles section, beginning on page 1.

SYNERGY BLENDS
Therapeutic-Quality Essential Oils
Combined to Enhance Their Effectiveness

Methods of use:

Intention: When using essential oils in subtle aromatherapy, they are used with intention. This simply means that you state, silently or aloud, the purpose for which you are using the essential oils and visualize the desired results.

Inhalation   Gentle Massage   Anointing

For more information, see Methods of Using Essential Oils on page xi.

NOTES

Depression
_____

Mix 12 drops Pick Me Up in 1 ounce of fractionated coconut oil or

fragrance-free, natural lotion. Massage feet and back.
_____

Foot Bath with 1 tablespoon Epsom salts and 2 drops Pick Me Up.
_____

Diffuse in room for family.
_____

Purification Odor Spray — mix 15-25 drops in 1 oz. spritzer bottle; fill with water.

Shake and spritz.
_____

_____

_____

_____

_____

_____

Hospice Solace

E3's Hospice Solace is designed to provide comfort and support. It was developed by a clinical aromatherapist with over fifteen years of experience in hospice settings.

The following essential oils are in **Hospice Solace** (alphabetical order). The therapeutic uses that are listed for each essential oil are those that are relevant to the purpose of this particular blend. In a hospice setting, the emotional and spiritual effects of essential oils may become especially important, and for this reason, the subtle aromatherapy uses are also listed.

Geranium: Immune support, stress, anxiety, mood swings, mild depression.
Subtle aromatherapy: Promotes harmony. Balances, comforts, uplifts, promotes a sense of peace, revitalizes, supports during times of change, soothes, nurtures.

Helichrysum: Muscle aches, immune support, mild depression, nervous exhaustion, shock.
Subtle aromatherapy: Clears energy blocks, promotes compassion for self and others, harmonizes, promotes meditative states, calms, promotes acceptance of change, strengthens, promotes patience and understanding.

Peppermint: Respiratory congestion, muscle spasms, mental fatigue, mental fog, nervous stress, mild depression.
Subtle aromatherapy: Promotes clarity in communication, inspires, awakens, encourages insights, refreshes, promotes self-acceptance.

Wintergreen: Muscle aches, muscle cramps, mental fog.
Subtle aromatherapy: Relaxes the logical mind, dispels resistance to change, promotes self-reflection.

Ylang Ylang Extra: Rapid breathing, tense breathing, general tension, stress, anxiety, sleeplessness, nervous tension, mild depression, anger, shock.
Subtle aromatherapy: Uplifts, promotes a sense of well-being, calms, soothes, promotes joy and enthusiasm.

For more information about the above, individual essential oils, please refer to the Singles section, beginning on page 1.

Methods of use:
Intention: When using essential oils in subtle aromatherapy, they are used with intention. This simply means that you state, silently or aloud, the purpose for which you are using the essential oils and visualize the desired results.

Inhalation   Gentle massage   Anointing

For more information, see Methods of Using Essential Oils on page xi.

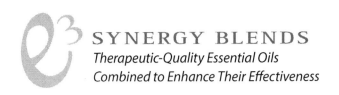

NOTES

Aches and pains

Mix 12 drops in 1 ounce of fractionated coconut oil or fragrance-free, natural lotion. Massage gently.

Hospice Transition

E3's Hospice Transition is designed to promote ease during times of change. It was developed by a clinical aromatherapist with over fifteen years of experience in hospice settings.

The following essential oils are in **Hospice Transition** (alphabetical order). The therapeutic uses that are listed for each essential oil are those that are relevant to the purpose of this particular blend. In a hospice setting, the emotional and spiritual effects of essential oils may become especially important, and for this reason, the subtle aromatherapy uses are also listed.

Bergamot, FCF: Mild depression, stress, anxiety, nervousness, mood swings, apathy.
Subtle aromatherapy: Brings in positive energy, eases grief, promotes acceptance, compassion, joy, balance, comfort and confidence.

Black Spruce: Stress, anxiety, mental fog.
Subtle aromatherapy: Clears and cleanses, promotes intuition, grounds, revitalizes, uplifts, promotes mental clarity and objectivity.

Frankincense: Tense breathing, rapid breathing, anxiety, stress, nervous tension, fear, restless mind.
Subtle aromatherapy: Quiets and clarifies the mind, calms, comforts, heals, promotes wisdom, focuses and strengthens spirituality, uplifts, promotes meditative states, stabilizes, promotes courage and strength, inspires, promotes acceptance.

Geranium: Stress, anxiety, mood swings, mild depression.
Subtle aromatherapy: Promotes harmony, balances, comforts, heals, uplifts, promotes a sense of peace, revitalizes, supports during times of change, soothes, nurtures.

Hyssop: Tense breathing, anxiety, tension, stress, mild depression, mental fog, inability to concentrate.
Subtle aromatherapy: Clears negativity, protects against influence of others' emotions, helps to ease grief.

Melissa: Rapid breathing, anxiety, mild depression, tension, crisis, fear, shock, anger.
Subtle aromatherapy: Uplifts, promotes understanding and acceptance, helps to ease grief, calms, promotes a sense of peace, strengthens, revitalizes, promotes happiness and cheerfulness.

Myrrh: Anxiety, tension, emotional coolness, apathy.
Subtle aromatherapy: Grounds, strengthens, supports spirituality, enhances visions, revitalizes, eases sorrow and grief, supports confident communication.

e³ SYNERGY BLENDS
Therapeutic-Quality Essential Oils
Combined to Enhance Their Effectiveness

Rose: Mild depression, stress, anxiety, irritability, tension, emotional coolness, sleeplessness, anger, fear.
Subtle aromatherapy: Brings in positive energy, promotes love and compassion, helps to release emotional wounds—especially grief, harmonizes, encourages forgiveness, comforts, promotes a sense of freedom and fulfillment.

Rosewood: Anxiety, stress, tension, mood swings, mild depression, emotional coolness.
Subtle aromatherapy: Brings in positive energy, clears energy blocks, promotes self-acceptance, gently opens the mind and heart.

Sandalwood: Anxiety, tension, stress, sleeplessness, sense of isolation, emotional instability.
Subtle aromatherapy: Calms, comforts, promotes the ability to trust and accept, supports insights and meditative states, promotes a sense of connectedness, balances, harmonizes, promotes wisdom and a sense of peace.

For more information about the above, individual essential oils, please refer to the Singles section, beginning on page 1.

Methods of use:
Intention: When using essential oils in subtle aromatherapy, they are used with intention. This simply means that you state, silently or aloud, the purpose for which you are using the essential oils and visualize the desired results.

Inhalation   Gentle massage   Anointing

For more information, see Methods of Using Essential Oils on page xi.

NOTES

For people adjusting to hospice care.

In the dying process to promote relaxation: Use as anointing oil on temples, forehead, behind ears, and on wrists. Mix 12 drops in 1 ounce of fractionated coconut oil or fragrance-free, natural lotion. Massage person's back and feet. (Massage chest if person likes it.)

e^3 *Dilutes*

PRECIOUS ESSENTIAL OILS
IN A 5% DILUTION

"Matter is the most spiritual
in the perfume of plants"

— Rudolph Steiner

Essential 3 has created Dilutes so that some of our precious essential oils can be enjoyed at a more affordable price. The essential oils or absolutes have been diluted in fractionated coconut oil. (Fractionated coconut oil does not go rancid, has no aroma of its own, and is non-greasy. For more information, see page 149.

E3 Dilutes may be applied directly to the skin and are ideal for use as therapeutics or natural perfumes.

Jasmine Dilute

Jasminum officinale var. grandiflorum
Aroma: Rich, warm, sweet, floral.
Extraction method: Absolute

Jasmine is an evergreen vine or shrub that is native to China and northern India. The delicate leaves are bright green, and the flowers are small, star-shaped, and exceptionally fragrant. The essential oil, extracted from the flowers, is prized for its sumptuous, intoxicating aroma and its aphrodisiac and euphoric properties. It is used extensively in perfumery and for psychological issues such as stress and mild depression.

For more information about Jasmine essential oil, please refer to page 39.

Helichrysum Dilute

Helichrysum italicum
Aroma: Spicy, rich, floral.
Extraction method: Steam distilled

Helichrysum is a common plant native to the Mediterranean. The name is derived from the Greek word "helios" meaning sun and "chrysos" meaning gold. The essential oil is distilled from the fragrant golden yellow flower heads; it is valued for its ability to decrease recovery time from small wounds, bruises and burns, calm nerve pain and reduce inflammation.

For more information about Helichrysum essential oil, please refer to page 38.

NOTES

Jasmine:
Aphrodisiac
Favorite perfume
Sleep aid

Helichrysum:
Unsurpassed for bruises
Calms nervous system

Melissa Dilute

Melissa officinalis
Aroma: Light, fresh, lemony.
Extraction method: Steam distilled

Melissa is a soft, bushy herb and is native to the Mediterranean area. It is also known as lemon balm or balm. The leaves have serrated edges and the tiny flowers are either white or pink. The essential oil, extracted from the whole plant, is prized for its use for viral infections, sleeplessness, and mild depression.

Neroli Dilute

Citrus aurantium
Aroma: Luxurious, sweet, slightly green-spicy, floral.
Extraction method: Steam distilled

The bitter orange tree is an evergreen that is native to the Far East and thrives in the Mediterranean area. It has dark green, oval-shaped, glossy leaves and small, wonderfully fragrant white flowers. This tree is unique in aromatherapy in that it produces three different essential oils: one from the leaves (petitgrain), one from the fruit (bitter orange), and one from the flowers (neroli or orange blossom). Neroli is one of the most treasured essential oils and is used for skin care, anxiety, and mild depression.

For more information about Neroli essential oil, please refer to page 53.

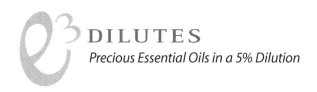

DILUTES
Precious Essential Oils in a 5% Dilution

Rose Dilute

also known as Rose Otto

Rosa damascena

Aroma: Elegant, feminine, refined, deep, spicy-sweet, floral.

Extraction method: Steam distilled

There are over 10,000 types of cultivated roses. The first cultivated rose is believed to be from Persia. Today, Morocco, Bulgaria, Turkey, and France are the primary growers of roses that are used for essential oil. Rose essential oil is extracted from the petals of the flowers and is cherished for its extensive use in perfumery, for its aphrodisiac properties, and for skin care. It is also used for psychological issues such as stress, emotional wounds, anxiety, and mild depression.

For more information about Rose essential oil, please refer to page 67.

Rose Dilute (Morocco)

Rosa centifolia

Aroma: Rich, feminine, spicy-sweet, floral.

Extraction method: Absolute

There are over 10,000 types of cultivated roses. The first cultivated rose is believed to be from Persia. Today, Morocco, Bulgaria, Turkey, and France are the primary growers of roses that are used for essential oil. Rose essential oil is extracted from the petals of the flowers and is cherished for its extensive use in perfumery, for its aphrodisiac properties, and for skin care. It is also used for psychological issues such as stress, emotional wounds, anxiety, and mild depression.

For more information about Rose, Morocco essential oil, please refer to page 68.

NOTES

Rose:

Stress relief

Skin care

Aphrodisiac

Sleep aid

Favorite perfume

Rose (Morocco):

Stress relief

Skin care

Aphrodisiac

Sleep aid

Favorite perfume

Carrier Oils

EMOLLIENT PLANT OILS

"The art of healing comes from nature,
not from the physician. Therefore the physician
must start from nature with an open mind."

— Paracelsus

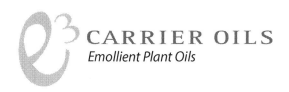

Fractionated Coconut Oil (FCO)

Cocos nucifera
Extraction method: Vacuum distilled
Storage: Highly stable, long shelf life.

Description:

Fractionated Coconut Oil (FCO) is a part or "fraction" of natural, whole coconut oil. FCO has had the long-chain triglycerides (fatty acids) separated and removed, leaving the medium-chain triglycerides. This separation is a physical, not chemical, process, so there are no undesirable chemical residues left behind.

FCO is an ideal carrier oil for aromatherapy uses and offers many benefits. It is odorless, clear, lightweight, non-greasy, easily absorbed, and highly stable (does not become rancid). It is also non-staining and can be washed out of fabric such as sheets and clothing.

FCO can be used alone or blended with other carrier oils for massage and skin care. It is good for all skin types to soothe, soften, and protect, and does not clog pores. It is also excellent as a base for perfumes and bath oils.

Basic Bath Oil

1 oz. FCO
25 drops of skin/bath-compatible essential oil (such as Lavender, Rose, Neroli, Frankincense, Chamomile).

Mix together and store in a small, glass bottle with a cap. Use 1 teaspoon per bath.

Basic Massage Oil #1

2 oz. FCO
12-24 drops of essential oil to suit the purpose of the massage.

Mix together and store in a small, glass bottle with a cap.

NOTES

All-purpose
Great bath oil
Long shelf life
Popular for massage

NOTES

Good for perfumes

Long shelf life

*Especially skin
  compatible*

Jojoba

Simmondsia chinensis

Extraction method: Cold pressed

Storage: Highly stable, long shelf life. May solidify in cooler temperatures. Remains fluid at room temperature.

Description:

Jojoba is extracted from the bean of a southwestern, evergreen, desert bush. Jojoba is more of a liquid wax than it is an oil. It is lightweight, non-greasy and easily absorbed. It is highly stable (resists rancidity) and has anti-inflammatory properties. It is especially compatible with skin because it closely resembles skin's natural oil, sebum, and does not clog pores.

Jojoba combines well at 25% with other carrier oils for massage, skin care, and scalp conditioning. It is good for all skin types to soothe, soften, and protect. It is often used alone as a base oil for perfumes.

Basic Perfume

1 T. Jojoba

10-20 drops of desired, skin-compatible essential oil (such as Jasmine or Rose)

Mix together and store in a small, glass bottle with a cap. Apply a drop to pulse points, such as the inner elbows, behind the knees, behind the ears, or on the underside of wrists.

Basic Massage Oil #2

1 oz. FCO

½ oz. Sweet Almond Oil

½ oz. Jojoba

12-24 drops of essential oil to suit the purpose of the massage.

Mix together and store in a small, glass bottle with a cap.

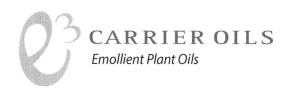

Rose Hip Seed Oil

Rosa mosqueta

Extraction method: Cold pressed

Storage: Keep refrigerated. Use within one year.

Description:

Rose Hip Seed Oil is cold-pressed from the tiny seeds of a South American, wild rose plant. It is a rich, emollient oil that penetrates well into the skin.

Rose Hip Seed Oil has been used for centuries by the Andean Indians to heal and care for the skin. Its regenerative properties have been attributed to its essential fatty acid content (linoleic and linolenic acids) and the presence of retinoic acid (a vitamin A derivative), which supports collagen production and cellular regeneration.

Rose Hip Seed Oil can be used alone or added (10% or more) to other products such as moisturizers, massage oils, or facial oils. It is used to soften fine lines and wrinkles, help repair sun-damaged skin, reduce scarring, improve elasticity, and protect the skin from environmental damage. It is helpful for dermatitis, sunburn, radiation burns, age spots, and stretch marks.

Basic Facial Oil #1

½ oz. Rose Hip Seed Oil
½ oz. FCO
2 drops Carrot Seed
2 drops Frankincense

Mix together and store in a small, glass bottle with a cap. To clean skin, apply about 5 drops and gently massage or pat.

Basic Scar / Stretch Mark Oil

1 T. Rose Hip Seed Oil
3 drops Helichrysum
2 drops Lavender, Spike

Mix together and store in a small, glass bottle with a cap. Apply a drop or two and gently massage.

NOTES

Regenerative

Scars

Sun-damage repair

Dermatitis

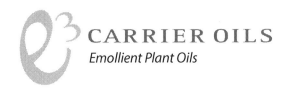

CARRIER OILS
Emollient Plant Oils

Popular for massage

Lightweight

Lubricating

Sweet Almond Oil

Prunis dulcis

Extraction method: Temperature controlled, low-resistance, expeller pressed

Storage: Keep refrigerated. Use within one year.

Description:

The sweet almond tree is native to the area from Asia to the Mediterranean. The oil is extracted from the nutmeats and is rich in vitamins and minerals. It is a lightweight oil that has excellent lubricating qualities, making it especially popular for massage.

Sweet Almond Oil can be used alone or blended with other carrier oils for massage and skin care. It is good for all skin types to soothe, soften, and protect and is helpful for dryness, itching, eczema, and dermatitis.

Basic Massage Oil #3

1 oz. FCO

1 oz. Sweet Almond Oil

12-24 drops of essential oil to suit the purpose of the massage.

Mix together and store in a small, glass bottle with a cap.

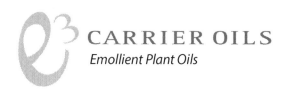

CARRIER OILS
Emollient Plant Oils

Tamanu

Calophyllum inophyllum
Extraction method: cold pressed, unrefined
Storage: Keep refrigerated. Use within one year.

Description:

The Calophyllum Inophyllum tree grows plentifully in the coastal regions of the South Pacific. (Its name means "beautiful leaf.") When its spherical fruit drop from the tree, they are collected, and cracked open. The kernel is removed and laid in the sun to dry. Over time, the kernels turn a deep-brown color and secrete a thick, rich, fragrant oil, which is cold-pressed from the kernel for use, and is called Tamanu.

(E3 sells only unrefined Tamanu, which is deeper in color, thicker, and richer in aroma and beneficial constituents than refined.)

Tamanu has been researched since the 1930s and has been used in hospitals for its wound-healing capabilities in Europe, Asia, and the Pacific Islands. It fights bacteria, reduces inflammation, and promotes the formation of new tissue. These capabilities are attributed to its unique content of lipids (neutral lipids, glycolipids, and phospholipids), calophyllic acid (a fatty acid), and calophyllolide (an anti-bacterial and non-steroidal anti-inflammatory).

Tamanu can be used alone or blended with other carrier oils. It is useful for insect bites, minor burns, small cuts, blisters, and scrapes. It is helpful for nerve pain conditions such as neuralgia, shingles, and sciatica. It also makes an excellent facial oil to smooth and soften the complexion.

NOTES

Smoothes and softens complexion

Dermatitis

Irritations

Nerve pain

Basic Facial Oil #2
½ oz. Tamanu
½ oz. FCO
2 drops Carrot Seed
2 drops Frankincense

Mix together and store in a small, glass bottle with a cap. To clean skin, apply about 5 drops and gently massage or pat.

Shingles Relief Oil
1 T. Tamanu
1 T. Ravensara

Mix together and store in a small, glass bottle with a cap. Apply directly to affected area several times a day as soon as symptoms begin. (Adapted from *Advanced Aromatherapy* by Dr. Kurt Schnaubelt.)

46071294R00101

Made in the USA
San Bernardino, CA
25 February 2017